PRAISE FOR *DEATH AND DOLLARS*

"For all those seeking a better understanding of why we rank last in healthcare outcomes of eleven industrialized nations, despite the trillions we spend, this book is a must-read."

CHRISTOPHER WHITE, M.D., ASSOCIATE MEDICAL
DIRECTOR, CHAIRMAN DEPARTMENT OF CARDIOLOGY,
OCHSNER HEALTH SYSTEM

"After an unflinching look at how we are failing to manage the chronic diseases of our time, Rich Milani tells us how connected patients and their data are about to reengineer the whole of US healthcare—every patient, clinician, and industry player should read this right now. "

DEBORAH KILPATRICK, PH.D., CEO,
EVIDATION HEALTH

"For anyone who wants to see the future of US Healthcare, read this powerful and visionary statement."

MICHAEL R. JAFF, D.O., PRESIDENT, NEWTON-
WELLESLEY HOSPITAL, PROFESSOR OF MEDICINE,
HARVARD MEDICAL SCHOOL

T0098609

"Dr. Milani writes about the epidemic of modern times—chronic disease. In an easy-to-read book, he dissects the components of this truly grand challenge. As a physician insider, Dr. Milani provides insights on how we got here and how we can transform our sick-care delivery organizations into health systems. Rich is an experienced, brilliant change agent! He explains how we can create the system Americans deserve—through culture, innovation, and social interventions. He explains how transformation is within our reach."

PAUL TANG, M.D., VICE PRESIDENT AND CHIEF TRANSFORMATION OFFICER, IBM WATSON HEALTH

"Dr. Richard Milani offers a new lens on the challenges of chronic disease, informed by his clinical work in New Orleans using digital health tools, better patient engagement, and big data analysis. Death and Dollars contains actionable insights for every public health official, hospital CEO, and med tech entrepreneur."

ZEN CHU, SENIOR LECTURER, MIT SLOAN SCHOOL OF MANAGEMENT AND FACULTY DIRECTOR, MIT HACKING MEDICINE INSTITUTE

Death *and* Dollars

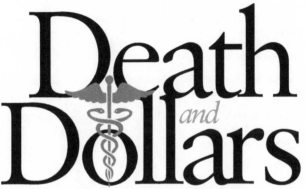

Death
and
Dollars

Solving the Epidemic of
CHRONIC DISEASE

Richard Milani, MD

NEW YORK

NASHVILLE • MELBOURNE • VANCOUVER

Death and Dollars

Solving the Epidemic of Chronic Disease

Published in New York, New York, by Morgan James Publishing. Morgan James is a trademark of Morgan James, LLC. www.MorganJamesPublishing.com

The Morgan James Speakers Group can bring authors to your live event. For more information or to book an event visit The Morgan James Speakers Group at www.TheMorganJamesSpeakersGroup.com.

ISBN 9781683505877 paperback
ISBN 9781683505884 eBook
Library of Congress Control Number: 2017907574

Cover Design by:
Rachel Lopez
www.r2cdesign.com

Interior Design by:
Chris Treccani
www.3dogcreative.net

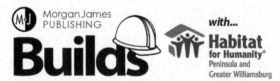

In an effort to support local communities, raise awareness and funds, Morgan James Publishing donates a percentage of all book sales for the life of each book to Habitat for Humanity Peninsula and Greater Williamsburg.

Get involved today! Visit
www.MorganJamesBuilds.com

TABLE OF CONTENTS

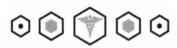

Chronic Disease Is an Epidemic and It's Killing Us

D r. Craig Spencer came down with a fever and gastrointestinal problems when he completed a medical mission in Guinea. His symptoms pointed to Ebola, a lethal virus that killed 11,284 people in the West African countries of Guinea, Sierra Leone, and Liberia in 2014 alone.[1] The thirty-three-year-old volunteer with Doctors Without Borders spent twenty days in a specially designed isolation unit at New York City's Bellevue Hospital. After

---

1   Centers for Disease Control, "2014 Ebola Outbreak in West Africa - Case Counts," www.cdc.gov/vhf/ebola/outbreaks/2014-west-africa/case-counts.html.

Spencer's healthcare team declared him virus-free, Mayor Bill de Blasio applauded Bellevue Hospital for implementing a perfectly executed treatment strategy that stopped the disease from infecting anybody else.

When it comes to fighting acute diseases and public health threats such as Ebola, the American healthcare system has few equals. A culture of innovation and product development has improved life measurably for millions of people. For at least seventy years, public and private funding have helped eradicate epidemics and acute disease that once shortened Americans' lives. Indeed, when HIV-AIDS began infecting and killing gay men in the early 1980s, medical researchers could largely rely on a scientific and governmental infrastructure to start working on a cure. In mid-1995, the U.S. Food and Drug Administration approved a three-drug cocktail that suppressed replication of the HIV virus. By 1996, the number of new AIDS cases diagnosed in the United States declined for the first time since the beginning of the epidemic.[2]

We take for granted that most of us will never suffer from acute diseases such as smallpox and polio. If we have access to regular medical care, we also no longer fear conditions that killed our parents and grandparents: hepatitis C, kidney infection, pneumonia, pancreatitis. We are all beneficiaries of the vaccines, drugs, and devices that have extended the lives of people suffering from infections and congenital heart disease.

---

2   AIDS.gov, "A Timeline of HIV/AIDS," www.aids.gov/hiv-aids-basics/hiv-aids-101/aids-timeline.

If you have to cope with an acute condition, better to live in 2015, not 1915.

But the healthcare narrative in America and other developed countries takes a different turn when we talk about chronic disease. Diabetes, hypertension, coronary heart disease, stroke, high cholesterol, gastric ulcers, arthritis, osteoporosis, chronic obstructive pulmonary disease, depression, and back pain are coming at us from every direction. Thirty percent of our health is genetic and we probably can't blame anything but our inherited biology. Most chronic disease, however, strikes us because of how we eat, how we spend our time, and how our healthcare system addresses our problems. In fact, medical researchers attribute 40 percent of our health to our behavioral patterns, 15 percent to social circumstances, 10 percent to healthcare, and 5 percent to environmental exposure.

Yet it's too easy to say that we are making ourselves sick. The 117 million Americans—about half of all adults—who have at least one chronic health condition are not totally to blame for overconsumption of foods high in sugar, salt and fat. Our supermarkets are temples to this stuff. Primary care doctors—the backbone of our healthcare system—aren't to blame for their patients' poor health either. As soon as they begin their clinical practice, doctors are overwhelmed by treating patients with six or seven chronic conditions in a ten- or fifteen-minute office visit. This schedule alone is a surefire recipe for poor health outcomes. Doctors don't have enough time to understand their patients' problems. They haven't been taught how to help patients actually change their behavior. They don't have an effective model to monitor patient progress.

Plus, they're expected to document every patient visit, comply with federal regulations, adhere to privacy laws and keep up with peer-reviewed papers on primary care topics.

When it comes to chronic disease, what is the central problem?

Patients and doctors alike participate in an outmoded healthcare system designed to treat acute disease—such as Ebola, heart attack, or upper respiratory infections, to name a few. The reality is that millions of us are struggling with chronic disease: obesity, diabetes, high cholesterol, high blood pressure, etc. Our healthcare system is simply not set up clinically, financially, or administratively to treat them.

We've known since 2001, when the Institute of Medicine, a division of the National Academies of Sciences, Engineering, and Medicine, reported that the delivery of care is "overly complex and uncoordinated, requiring steps and patient 'handoffs' that slow down care and decrease rather than improve safety."[3] We can all attest to the IOM's diagnosis. Like many twentieth-century systems, our healthcare organizations, medical centers and physician groups function as separate silos. A patient's cardiologist and neurologist probably don't know of each other's existence. It's as if the Internet technologies that dramatically transformed our economy over the past twenty years have had little impact on the healthcare industry at all.

---

3   Institute of Medicine, "Crossing the Quality Chasm: A New Health System for the 21st Century," March 2001, https://iom. nationalacademies.org/~/media/Files/Report%20Files/2001/Crossing-the-Quality-Chasm/Quality%20Chasm%202001%20%20report%20 brief.pdf.

Maintaining a badly functioning healthcare system has had severe consequences on our personal health and on the health of our society. In 2013, the year for which we have the most recent data, the United States spent $2.9 trillion on healthcare, or about $9,255 per person.[4] That's tantamount to 17.4 percent of Gross Domestic Product (GDP). By 2024, the healthcare share of GDP is expected to rise to 19.6 percent.

There's no lack of mind-blowing statistics on the amount of money that we—households, governments, private business and other entities—spend every year on healthcare. For all the trillions we're spending, though, shouldn't we rank higher than eleventh of eleven industrialized nations when it comes to healthcare outcomes? A Commonwealth Fund study found that we're also last or near last on health system quality, efficiency, access to care, and equity. By comparison, the United Kingdom, which spent $3,406 per capita in 2011, ranked first on the same metrics based largely on national mortality data (although it too lagged on health outcomes).[5]

The data show a great disconnect between the money spent on healthcare and outcomes: of that $2.9 trillion spent on

---

4   Centers for Medicare & Medicaid Services, "National Health Expenditure Fact Sheet,"www.cms.gov/Research-Statistics-Data-and-Systems/Statistics-Trends-and-Reports/NationalHealthExpendData/NHE-Fact-Sheet.html.

5   The World Bank, "Health Expenditure Per Capita (current US$)," http://data.worldbank.org/indicator/SH.XPD.PCAP.

healthcare, $2.5 trillion, or 86 percent of all healthcare spending, goes to treating patients with one or more chronic diseases.[6]

So, how's this system working out for us?

Not so good. Chronic disease is responsible for seven out of every ten deaths in the United States (as of 2010). Heart disease, cancer, stroke, diabetes, kidney disease, and other chronic conditions kill more than 1.7 million Americans every year.[7]

Primary care doctors—the first responders in the chronic disease epidemic—can tell you that their middle-aged and older patients are coming in sick with diabetes or pre-diabetes and high cholesterol; and their young patients—roughly one in six children between six and nineteen—are overweight.[8] You cannot see a steady stream of chronically sick patients, month after month, year after year, and feel that you are truly helping people get healthy. In fact, only 36 percent of physicians are satisfied with the care they give these patients—as compared

---

6   In the United States, $1.65 trillion, or 75 percent of all healthcare spending, goes to treating patients with one or more chronic disease. The annual economic impact on the U.S. of the seven most common chronic diseases is about $1.3 trillion. This figure could balloon to nearly $6 trillion by 2050. Partnership to Fight Chronic Disease, "Fighting Chronic Disease: The Case for Enhancing the Congressional Budget Analysis Process," www.fightchronicdisease. org/sites/fightchronicdisease.org/files/docs/PFCD_ChronDisease_ FactSheet3Final.pdf.

7   Centers for Disease Control and Prevention, "Chronic Disease Prevention and Health Promotion," http://www.cdc.gov/ chronicdisease/overview.

8   Partnership to Fight Chronic Disease, "The Growing Crisis of Chronic Disease in the United States," http://www. fightchronicdisease.org/sites/fightchronicdisease.org/files/docs/ GrowingCrisisofChronicDiseaseintheUSfactsheet_81009.pdf.

to 54 percent who are satisfied with the care they give their general patients.

What primary care physicians also recognize is that the prescription pad is a limited healthcare tool. For every individual helped by the ten highest-grossing drugs in the United States to control cholesterol, diabetes, asthma, Crohn's disease, arthritis, and other chronic conditions, between three and twenty-five people report no benefit at all.[9]

An equally serious problem is the lack of patient adherence. Medical researchers in 2011 learned that even when medications are effective in combating disease, their full benefits are not realized because some fifty percent of patients don't take their medications as prescribed.[10] Once again it makes no sense to blame the patient. Who wants somebody to shove a prescription down their throat and say, "Take this drug or else! Scaring people into going straight has never worked and never will.

If you're on a leaky ship, putting up a new mast won't keep it from taking on more water. Likewise, a new insurance carrier or a new low-level "care manager" is not going to reverse the physiological, social, psychological, financial, and organizational deficits spawned by chronic disease. A healthcare system that cannot prevent 1.7 million new diagnoses of diabetes a year or help contain the $245 billion for the total cost of the disease

---

9   The Chronic Disease Center of Excellence | Healthcare Focus Factory, p. 48.

10   Marie T. Brown and Jennifer K. Bussell, "Medication Adherence: WHO Cares?" *Mayo Clinic Proceedings* 86, no. 4 (April 2011): 304–14, http://www.ncbi.nlm.nih.gov/pmc/articles/PMC3068890.

in diagnosed patients alone is a system that is listing toward an unsustainable future.[11] Writing out more prescriptions, warning people that smoking is bad for you, restricting wellness visits to once a year to keep healthcare costs down, certifying support staff as chronic disease case managers—trying harder in these ways to change individuals and systems isn't much of a solution at all.

A system that should be keeping us healthy is keeping us sick.

I have seen this assertion borne out in my own practice as a cardiologist.

Eighty percent of the cardiovascular conditions I have observed as vice chairman of the department of cardiology in the Ochsner Health System in New Orleans, and as Ochsner's chief clinical transformation officer, stem not only from unhealthy lifestyle habits, but also from a perverse systemic approach to disease prevention. What typically happens is you or a loved one comes to us after having a heart attack. Once we've got you stabilized, you enter into a three-month rehabilitation program consisting of exercise and education three times a week. We'll "teach" you about your risk factors that led to your heart attack such as smoking, poor diet, or lack of exercise. You'll also join a cohort of patients with the same health and lifestyle problems you have. You'll exercise for 30 minutes on the treadmill or elliptical. We'll put you on a healthier diet—and presto

---

11   American Diabetes Association, "Statistics about Diabetes," www. diabetes.org/diabetes-basics/statistics.

change-o—you'll leave a more enlightened and changed man or woman.

This well-intentioned therapeutic plan has two flaws: First, many of you will likely resume the very habits that gave you a heart attack or stroke in the first place. Not because you're bad or weak-willed, but because you no longer have the support of your group. Second, you can't stick with the program because we've compelled you to participate in a cart-before-the-horse plan. We should have enrolled you in a cardiac health program one year ago. But who in the American healthcare system reimburses you for preventive care? We'll spend billions of dollars on you after you get sick, but not before when we can really help you. Sadly, the only behavior-change tool we have in our healthcare doctor's bag is too little too late.

A hopeless situation, right?

It's not!

The Internet of Things—the connection of devices to the Internet and to each other—has given us an arsenal of behavior-change tools. Wearable technology, like a Fitbit, theoretically could help your primary care physician infer from weekly, monthly, or quarterly data why your cholesterol or blood pressure is high.

At Ochsner we initiated a hypertension digital medicine program in April 2015 that uses an Apple Watch, as well as other wireless devices, to help patients measure their blood pressure and heart rate at home. The numbers are sent automatically to Ochsner clinical pharmacists and health coaches so that they—not low-level "care managers"—can inform patients about necessary medication or lifestyle adjustments. Patients also get medication reminders, clinical feedback, prescription renewals, activity trackers and other relevant information. Best of all, we have data to show that patients and doctors are benefiting from our program, primarily because that data is continuous. We're not just looking episodically at information we gather three or four times a year during short office visits.

We have to talk about a reformed healthcare system that can respond almost instantly to patients before they suffer a heart attack or stroke—a system that may even reduce the number of times patients have to come in for a check-up. Fewer appointments also reduce daily patient caseload, freeing up physicians' schedules to handle other patients in need.

I don't want to minimize the complexity that accompanies digital data collection. We have to ensure patient privacy. We have to work with insurance companies so they don't use personal data to penalize patients or doctors. But the potential benefits of patient-generated health data are too great to dismiss. Technology is valuable because it lets patients interact with each other as well as with their physicians. Sustainable changes in patient behavior do not come from me telling a patient what to do. They come about in a dynamic way when technology helps human beings learn tactics and strategies about themselves and from each other. As Ben Franklin once said: "Tell me and I forget. Teach me and I may remember. Involve me and I learn."

● ⬡ ●

I started this chapter by talking about Ebola, an extreme disease as similar to chronic disease as laser tag is to hopscotch.

But chronic disease and Ebola actually have something in common with each other. They are both communicable diseases. Research shows that if you associate with people who make unhealthy food choices, you're likely to make those same choices.[12] Connecting with people similar to you, in real life and on social networks, appears to force less-healthy individuals to interact primarily with one another. The people most in need of a health innovation that could alter their behavior may be among the least likely to adopt it.

Yet some studies show that in certain controlled situations, people with the same social contacts can be influenced to adopt a new health behavior.[13] Anecdotally speaking, we see that happen all the time in online and real-world support groups. Even if it turns out that there's a genetic component underlying the tendency for obese people, for example, to cluster in large social networks, we now have technologies that will let us investigate the legitimacy of this assertion.[14]

---

12 Hristina Dzhogleva and Cait Poynor Lamberton, "Should Birds of a Feather Flock Together? Understanding Self-Control Decisions in Dyads," *Journal of Consumer Research* 41, no. 2 (August 2014): 361-80, http://jcr.oxfordjournals.org/content/41/2/361.

13 Damon Centola, "An Experimental Study of Homophily in the Adoption of Health Behavior," *Science* 334, no. 6060 (December 2011): 1269–72, www.sciencemag.org/content/334/6060/1269.short.

14 Kenneth Blum et al., "Neuropsychiatric Genetics of Happiness, Friendships, and Politics: Hypothesizing Homophily ("Birds of a Feather Flock Together") as a Function of Reward Gene Polymorphisms," Journal of Genetic Syndromes & Gene Therapy 3, no. 112 (April 2012), www.ncbi.nlm.nih.gov/pmc/articles/PMC3547641.

Healthcare organizations, such as the Centers for Disease Control, the World Health Organization and numerous nongovernmental organizations understood (some right away, some eventually) that letting Ebola run its course could result in the deaths of thousands, perhaps hundreds of thousands, of people. Poorly managed chronic disease is having a comparable, albeit less sensational, impact on millions of people in the United States and elsewhere.

We already know a lot about the root causes of our chronic disease epidemic. We know the bad news:

- Chronic disease is responsible for 86 percent of healthcare costs and the majority of deaths in the United States.
- Existing delivery models are poorly constructed to manage chronic disease, as evidenced by low adherence to quality and control indicators.
- But we know the good news too:
- New technologies have emerged that can engage patients and offer additional modalities in treating chronic disease.
- Modifying healthcare delivery to include team-based care combined with patient-centered technologies offers great promise.

In the next ten chapters, I'll talk about how each one of us (physicians, administrators and policy makers), must help our patients become active partners in their own healthcare. Thanks in part to smart phone apps, wearable technology and home devices, we can make this happen. Popular technologies and structural fixes in our healthcare delivery system give us the power to design a cost-effective nonpharmacological scheme that will encourage people to change their negative behaviors. I believe that a reengineered healthcare system has the power to extend people's lives.

What do we do first?

For starters, we have to stop blaming the patient and the primary care physician for systemic problems that put all kinds of strain on patients, families, hospitals, and workplaces.

Next we have to transform the current care delivery model so that we can manage chronic disease—the medical crisis of the twenty-first century. The model we develop must include integrated units of pharmacists, advanced practice clinicians, nurses, health educators, dietitians, social workers, counselors, and therapists who can competently take up the job of managing chronic disease where the physician has to leave off.

Finally, the healthcare industry has to avail itself of the same just-in-time technologies that have reshaped other sectors of the economy. These will put people in touch with each other, deliver services at the tap of an app, and lower the cost of delivering care.

This country is facing huge challenges in education, homeland security, cybersecurity, climate change, employment, and infrastructure. We can't afford to be distracted by diseases that we can prevent. We can't afford to tax a shrinking workforce population of millennials, Gen Xers, and baby boomers so that we can keep putting Band-Aids on a societal wound that needs major surgery. A healthy healthcare system isn't just a nice to have. It's a need to have.

When you come to a fork in the road, take it.

That's where we've got to start.

CHAPTER 1

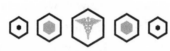

Fighting a 21st-Century Problem with a 19th-Century Healthcare System

W hen Edwin Starr asked and answered his own question—"War, what is it good for?" "Absolutely nothing!"—he was, sadly, mistaken. The Crimean War (1853–56) and the American Civil War (1861–65) served as incubators for an acute civilian healthcare system that came to include ambulance service, the credentialing of doctors and nurses, triage decision-making and surgery, and palliative care. The patient, who arrived via ambulance to a late nineteenth-century municipal hospital, received the optimal care of the day for appendicitis, angina pectoris, pneumonia, diarrhea, catarrh, tuberculosis, gastritis, peritonitis, and a raft of other acute conditions.[15] Indeed, the first official hospitals were designed to address the episodic nature of disease. By and large, acute care improved further with the arrival in the twentieth century of antibiotics, disinfectants, and vaccines.

The acute healthcare framework was one of the great social innovations of the mid-to-late nineteenth century, and many of us are here today because our ancestors were spared premature death from an acute disease. Despite continued advances in medical care, though, the death rate per 100,000 people began to climb in 1950. Neurasthenia and apoplexy now gave way to chronic conditions such as heart disease, cancer, diabetes, pulmonary disease, and cerebrovascular disease. Primarily lifestyle diseases, they were the result of the food we ate and the air we breathed. They also arose out of a culturally sanctioned message to sit (watch TV and eat processed food) instead of move (exercise or go for a walk).

The chronic diseases that began in the mid-1950s and peaked in the late 1960s, remain with us today. And unlike acute diseases, which can be treated by setting a broken bone or prescribing an antibiotic, chronic conditions result in the patient's steady decline into debilitating—and economically draining—illness. Healthcare economists across the ideological spectrum increasingly recognize the folly of using an anachronistic acute healthcare system to deal with diseases that

---

15   Karin L. Flippin, "Causes of Death in the Late 19th Century Mentioned in the Register of Deaths, 1893–1907," April 1997, http:// courses.wcupa.edu/jones/his480/notes/deth-dic.htm.

may begin as early as childhood and extend into middle and old age.

What we have today is a healthcare model adapted to the health needs of people in the late nineteenth century. Little wonder that it is failing patients, families, providers, medical centers, workplaces, and society in the twenty-first century.

It's not as if our country is ignoring chronic disease. According to official U.S. estimates, healthcare spending in 2014 reached $2.9 trillion.16 By 2024, it's projected to hit $5.4 trillion—19.6 percent of the gross domestic product (GDP). The system designed to treat a fall from a horse and buggy (and a host of other serious one-time events) today spends $1.224 billion for treating heart disease, $421 million for coronary heart disease, $1.011 billion for diabetes, and $107 million for COPD.17

How's all that expenditure working out for us?

Not so good.

Seven of every ten deaths in the United States are caused by chronic conditions. Heart disease is the leading cause of death among men and women, followed by cancer and chronic obstructive pulmonary diseases. Diabetes ranks seventh.[18]

---

16 Cynthia Cox, "Health Spending Growth Expected to Bounce Back in Coming Years," updated August 11, 2015, http://www. healthsystemtracker.org/2015/07/health-spending-growth-expected-to-bounce-back-in-coming-years.

17 National Institute of Health, "Estimates of Funding for Various Research, Condition, and Disease Categories (RCDC)," February 10, 2016, http://report.nih.gov/categorical_spending.aspx.

18 National Conference of State Legislatures, October 2012, www.ncsl.org/research/health/chronic-disease-prevention-and-health-promotion.aspx.

To be fair, outcomes aren't always disappointing. The Milken Institute, which recently updated its 2007 study on the cost of chronic disease and wellness in America, reports that treatment expenditures per patient and heart disease prevalence in 2013 were lower than the Institute's baseline projections. In all other chronic diseases, however, patients reporting a chronic condition rose *beyond* baseline projections—and actual treatment costs and productivity losses *exceeded* estimates.[19]

Despite the guardedly optimistic news about heart disease, chronic illness nonetheless affects one of every two adults in the United States.[20] It's responsible for a staggering 80 percent of all healthcare costs.[21] With healthcare spending up in the stratosphere, and with many well-intentioned campaigns emphasizing the role of diet and exercise in maintaining good health, why are so many Americans chronically sick?

Let's first establish an accurate definition of chronic disease. The World Health Organization categorizes it as a noncommunicable disease (NCD) that kills 38 million people each year. The WHO offers a mortality breakdown of each NCD—cardiovascular diseases, cancers, respiratory diseases,

---

19   Anusuya Chatterjee, Sindhu Kubendran, Jaque King, and Ross DeVol, "Measuring the Economic Burden in a Changing Nation," Checkup Time: Chronic Disease and Wellness in America (The Milken Institute, 2014), http://assets1b.milkeninstitute.org/assets/Publication/ResearchReport/PDF/Checkup-Time-Chronic-Disease-and-Wellness-in-America.pdf.

20   Chatterjee et al., "Measuring the Economic Burden in a Changing Nation," *Checkup Time: Chronic Disease and Wellness in America.*

21   "The Chronic Disease Center of Excellence: A New Paradigm for Healthcare Delivery."

and diabetes)—and links all four groups to tobacco use, physical inactivity, the harmful use of alcohol, and unhealthy diets.[22] GlobalHealth.gov, state.gov, the European Commission, and other agencies and nongovernmental organizations concur: chronic disease is a noncommunicable condition that represents "leading causes of mortality."[23]

They've all got it wrong.

With chronic disease, we are dealing with noninfectious conditions that nonetheless are *communicable* across populations. And while chronic illness is principally due to four self-activated behaviors—physical inactivity, poor nutrition, tobacco use, and excess alcohol consumption—these behaviors escalate when friends and acquaintances interact with each other. Physicians and public health researchers have even found that these and other contributing health behaviors, such as medication adherence, represent an interpersonal contagion with measurable impact up to three degrees of influence within social networks. Using "network statistics," for example, social scientists Nicholas A. Christakis and James H. Fowler examined several data sets, including the Framingham Heart Study and the National Longitudinal Study of Adolescent Health, to observe the spread of obesity, smoking, heavy drinking, and drug use

---

22   World Health Organization Media Centre, "Noncommunicable Diseases," updated January 2015, www.who.int/mediacentre/factsheets/fs355/en.

23   http://www.globalhealth.gov/global-health-topics/non-communicable-diseases; U.S. Department of State, "Infectious and Chronic Disease," www.state.gov/e/oes/intlhealthbiodefense/id; and European Commission, "Major and Chronic Diseases," http://ec.europa.eu/health/major_chronic_diseases/policy/index_en.htm.

along interpersonal pathways. (Our good habits—cooperative behavior, political mobilization, and tastes in music, books, and movies—proceed along the same pathways.) Christakis, Fowler, and a growing school of like-minded researchers found that, in order to advance good health outcomes, healthcare systems must also pay attention to the relatives, friends, and colleagues that make up a patient's social network.[24] One set of researchers concluded that the "distal elements of personal social relationships," say, a patient's Facebook friends, can help reduce healthcare costs by 50 percent simply by "being there" for the patient.[25]

Healthcare delivery systems need to be designed with the awareness that we are all social animals. The choices we make about diet, alcohol, drugs, and exercise are influenced by our subjective biases, habits, and social norms. Rather than focus exclusively on the doctor-patient relationship, healthcare systems have to develop a supportive ecosystem that acknowledges the *communicability* of chronic disease. They have

---

24   "The Chronic Disease Center of Excellence: A New Paradigm for Healthcare Delivery." See also Nicholas A. Christakis and James H. Fowler, "Social Contagion Theory: Examining Dynamic Social Networks and Human Behavior," *Statistics in Medicine* 32, no. 4 (February 2013): 556–77, www.ncbi.nlm.nih.gov/pmc/articles/PMC3830455.

25   "The Chronic Disease Center of Excellence: A New Paradigm for Healthcare Delivery." See also David Reeves, Christian Blickem, Ivaylo Vassilev, Helen Brooks, Anne Kennedy, Gerry Richardson, and Anne Rogers, "The Contribution of Social Networks to the Health and Self-Management of Patients with Long-Term Conditions: A Longitudinal Study," PLoS ONE 9, no. 6 (June 2014), http://journals.plos.org/plosone/article?id=10.1371/journal.pone.0098340.

to engage patients and their social networks to work toward healthier lifestyle habits. As challenging as this may sound, it's actually simpler—and cheaper—than intervening in a patient's life when she is already experiencing kidney, heart, and lung failure due to a host of runaway chronic diseases.

A second problem concerns how chronic disease itself is managed. If treating diabetes, for example, was a matter of undergoing a one-time operation, or getting a one-time injection of insulin, the acute care system would still be eminently workable, at least for this disease. But diabetics have a lot on their plate, so to speak. They have to observe a diet low in calories, simple carbohydrates and saturated fat, a strict exercise regimen and a balanced intake of insulin and oral medications. Due to the nature of the disease, blood sugar levels can yo-yo up and down. These changes may be slight or severe, but they are near-constant. Yet many physicians are still seeing their diabetic patients only three or four times a year. Despite the physician's best efforts, episodic treatment of diabetes can result in an acute condition requiring a heart procedure such as a stent, pancreas transplant, or an amputation.

Nobody would choose these outcomes if they had a better choice.

The better choice exists.

Digital technologies have put all kinds of activities— shopping, dating, banking, hailing, learning, *and disease monitoring*—into everybody's hands. We're not talking about some Jetsons-like future. The Fitbit and the Apple Watch, two of the most popular patient monitoring devices, are already improving healthcare outcomes just as antibiotics did a century ago.[26] Lots of other game-changing health products are on the horizon too:

- An ear bud tracker to monitor real-time blood pressure, respiration rate, oxygen saturation, heart rate, calories burned, and steps. Some trackers are able to monitor your eating habits and "nudge" you to eat more slowly, eat less or drink more water.
- A sweat sensor strip that measures the metabolic substances secreted in your sweat. It tracks electrolyte balance, hydration level, muscle exertion, and physical performance—insights that surpass what we can learn from steps and heart rate alone.
- A smartphone case that doubles as an electrocardiograph machine and a DIY blood tester. The patient holds an FDA-approved iPhone case, and thirty seconds later, he can send his doctor an ECG and plausibly take action to prevent a stroke.

These tracking devices are powerful because they collect a steady stream of physiological data that the patient can share with his healthcare provider. A doctor, nurse, dietician, physical therapist or wellness coach can respond within hours or minutes.

The office visit of the twenty-first century, then, takes place via wearable technology and a smartphone. The patient can send in his data from home, workplace, school, or gym. Most

---

26   Leyl Master Black, "5 Digital Health Trends You'll See in 2015," www. cnn.com/2014/12/19/tech/partner-digital-health-trends.

important, he doesn't have to wait for a doctor's appointment, because a member of his integrated healthcare team can respond faster at lower cost. As for the physician, her schedule has been freed up to deal with urgent and emergency cases.

We have evidence that the digital office visit works.

In 2014, the Ochsner Health System combined the Epic Electronic Health Record (EHR) system and Apple Health, a healthcare data-sharing mobile app, to evaluate heart failure hospital readmissions, a common problem for patients with congestive heart failure.[27] Post-hospitalization, patients went home with a wireless scale that transmitted relevant data to their Ochsner physician and a clinical pharmacist. Ochsner was able to track the relationship between fluid retention and weight gain and then alert the patient by phone to adjust their medication accordingly. As a result, hospital readmissions were reduced by 45 percent and patients were able to be at home or work instead of being in a hospital bed.

Ochsner also evaluated patients who had out-of-control hypertension. Patients were monitored from their home using a wireless blood pressure cuff integrated into Apple's HealthKit. The cuff was easy to use and patient adherence was high due to the convenience of managing their chronic condition from home. Healthcare teams collected robust data and shared it with patients. They also engaged patients in a mutually agreed upon

27   David Harlow, "Apple HealthKit – Epic Integration at Ochsner Health System – David Harlow Interviews Dr. Richard Milani," HealthBlawg, October 14, 2014, http://healthblawg.com/2014/10/apple-healthkit-epic-integration-at-ochsner-health-system-david-harlow-interviews-dr-richard-milani.html.

plan to increase exercise and/or change their diet, with the goal of reducing high blood pressure. Within a short period of time, patients saw that lifestyle changes in combination with better medical management helped lower blood pressure to target goals. For patients who wanted more granular information, the therapeutic team offered a lab report visualization. Take a look at Illustration 1 to see how color-coded diagrams give patients lifesaving information at a glance.

Hypertension Digital Medicine Report
Test Patient

What is High Blood Pressure?

High blood pressure, also called hypertension, occurs when the pressure inside your arteries is higher than it should be. One in three American adults has high blood pressure, and if it is not controlled, it can cause damage to your eyes, brain, heart, blood vessels and kidneys; as a result, high blood pressure is a leading cause of heart attack and stroke. High blood pressure has no warning signs or symptoms, so monitoring your blood pressure readings and getting it under control is very important to your health and well-being.

Your Results   Excellent ☺

Systolic

138

<90	90-139	140-180	>180
Low	Desired	High	Danger

Diastolic

87

<60	60-89	90-110	>110
Low	Desired	High	Danger

Your Progress

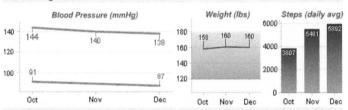

Blood Pressure (mmHg) — 144, 140, 138 / 91, 87 — Oct, Nov, Dec

Weight (lbs) — 158, 160, 160 — Oct, Nov, Dec

Steps (daily avg) — 3807, 5481, 5892 — Oct, Nov, Dec

Your Risk

With your current medical conditions, the 10 year estimated risk of heart attack and stroke is: **16%**

You can reduce your risk to:
10% if your blood pressure was 120 mm/Hg
6% if your HDL cholesterol was at least 60 mg/dL

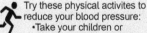

Try these physical activites to reduce your blood pressure:
- Take your children or grandchildren to the park.
- Take a 30-minute window-shopping walk around the mall when weather is bad.

Did you know that the more alcohol you drink, the higher your blood pressure? The good news is that by reducing your alcohol intake, ideally to less than 2 alcoholic drinks per day, you can effectively lower blood pressure.

Illustration 1

We have evidence of a link between wearable and/or home-based technology and improved healthcare outcomes at other healthcare delivery organizations too. A case in point is CareMore, a for-profit, privately held corporation whose patient base of chronically ill members (approximately 15 percent) accounts for 70 percent of medical costs. In one study (2011) at the office in Downey, California, CareMore nurse practitioners saw hundreds of network members—average age 72, Hispanic (45 percent), diabetic (34 percent), hypertensive (40 percent), and living on an annual income of $30,000 or less (50 percent). The nurses used several examining rooms to see patients, but the heartbeat of the place was a warren of rooms filled with computer monitors and phone banks. Here the nurse practitioners and medical assistants relied on EHRs, an integrated view of pharmacy, laboratory and utilization data, and remote wireless technology to monitor patients' chronic conditions: heart failure, end-stage renal disease, kidney disease, COPD, hypertension, mental health disorders, anticoagulation, diabetes mellitus, and wound care, falls, palliative care, and hospice.[28]

If the tech-dependent CareMore healthcare delivery model seems like a We-Could-Care-Less model, consider the healthcare outcomes:

- Elderly patients with diabetes mellitus had an average glycosylated hemoglobin level of 7.08 and

---

28   David B. Reuben, "Physicians in Supporting Roles in Chronic Disease Care: The CareMore Model," *Journal of the American Geriatrics Society* 59, no. 1 (January 2011): 158–60.

an amputation rate 78 percent less than the national average.

- Hospitalizations for end-stage renal disease were 42 percent less than the national average.
- Thirty-day rehospitalization rates were 13.6 percent, compared with 20 percent in the overall Medicare population.

Wondering if the patients got insufficient care?

Patients gave CareMore an 8.81 out of 10 rating (2009). The national average patient satisfaction rating was 8.47; the California state average 8.57.

It must have cost a fortune.

It didn't.

CareMore estimated that payers' risk-adjusted total per capita health spending was 15 percent below the regional average. The corporation accomplished its goal to "protect precious financial resources of seniors and the Medicare Program through innovative methods of managing chronic disease, frailty, and end of life" even while forgoing copayments and deductibles. CareMore also offered members no-cost transportation services to its centers, free three-month membership in "Nifty After Fifty" fitness centers, podiatry care, house calls by physicians and nurse practitioners, an intervention team that investigated nonclinical problems in patients' homes, caregiver support, respite care, and a high-intensity management program for the frailest patients.

CareMore has remained highly profitable.

A healthcare delivery system with an emphasis on managing chronic disease through dynamic technology systems and an integrated healthcare team is financially responsible and effective.

Ochsner and CareMore are both regional healthcare networks. Can a digitally based system scale to meet the demands of a national system?

The Centers for Medicare & Medicaid Services (CMS) spending growth rates rose 5.9 percent (2000-2008), 1.8 percent (2009-2012), and a negligible 0.2 percent in 2013. The slowdown in spending over this period is due partly to a reduction in utilization: Medicare patients are using the healthcare system less intensely than they did in the early to mid 2000s. This may be good or bad, depending on the reasons for the drop-off. What's interesting here is that changes to Medicare reimbursement rates are also helping the system save money.

In October 2012, CMS instituted Value-Based Purchasing (VBP), an initiative that rewards acute-care hospitals with incentive payments for the quality—not quantity—of care they provide to people with Medicare.[29] In its first year, the VBP initiative assessed the clinical process and patient experience. By 2014 it was also able to look at health outcomes. In 2015 it added an efficiency metric. Because all metrics improved over time, acute-care hospitals were rewarded applicable percentages

---

29   Department of Health & Human Services, CMS, "Hospital Value-Based Purchasing,"www.cms.gov/Outreach-and-Education/Medicare-Learning-Network-MLN/MLNProducts/Downloads/Hospital_VBPurchasing_Fact_Sheet_ICN907664.pdf.

ranging from 1.0 percent (2013) to 1.5 percent (2015). Rewards are expected to climb to 2.0 percent beginning in 2017.

Of course, the CMS assessment of VBP focused exclusively on acute episodic conditions, including acute myocardial infarction, acute heart failure, pneumonia, and other conditions. But if the incentive program could improve healthcare quality and quality of care in the inpatient hospital setting, why can't a comparable program do the same for chronic care?

We need a VBP-style healthcare model that rewards physicians and other providers for practicing medicine that keeps patients out of the hospital, enhances patient satisfaction, and increases healthy outcomes. The fee-for-service paradigm, which rewards physicians for number of tasks performed, is a payment mechanism that will hamstring even the best high-tech healthcare management program. Tying payments to patient outcomes instead of to services rendered will result in substantial savings and a healthier population.

The $315.9 billion that CMS cut out of Medicare spending? Sixty-nine billion of it could have funded the Children's Health Insurance Program (CHIP), $15 billion the National Park Service, and $7 billion Amtrak. The remaining $53 billion would have paid for all the movie tickets sold between 2009 and 2013. Now multiply these funds and revenues twice—and you'll have the total of Medicare's savings in the performance period.30

---

30   Christophe Haubursin, "Medicare Just Saved More Than 10 Times the Combined Cost of Amtrak and the National Parks," www.vox.com/2015/4/16/8424139/medicare-just-saved-more-than-10-times-the-combined-cost-of-amtrak.

Physicians, insurers, healthcare systems and patients see firsthand the consequences of applying a nineteenth-century acute care system to twenty-first century chronic disease. If that's the case, why don't we see a healthcare system that serves the health needs of its patients?

We have to reach a tipping point before providers, payers, and consumers agitate for a system that will take on the diseases that are killing our family, friends, and coworkers.

That tipping point may come only with an increase in deaths of people who can't afford the car fare to see their doctor, or when millions of people suffer from multiple chronic diseases because they believe fast food can substitute for a wholesome meal.

It may come when the average cost per inpatient day at an American non-profit hospital is $2,289, $1,791 at a for-profit hospital, and $1,878 at a state or local government hospital.31

It may come when the Internet of Things is so pervasive in our lives that it makes no sense for the healthcare industry to be off the grid.

We're there.

[As author William Gibson said: "The future is already here—it's just not very evenly distributed."]

---

31   Emily Rappleye, "Average Cost Per Inpatient Day Across 50 States," http://www.beckershospitalreview.com/finance/average-cost-per-inpatient-day-across-50-states.html.

CHAPTER 2

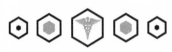

Behavior Is
Communicable–and We
Can Prove It

B ack before the digital revolution, physicists and other
natural scientists tended to dismiss psychology, sociology
and economics as the "soft sciences." No matter that
the practitioners of these three "intuitive" disciplines sought to
apply the scientific method to their analysis of individual and
group behavior. Natural scientists, who rely on quantifiable data
and mathematical models, typically deemed the observations
of social scientists as interesting but anecdotal. It probably
didn't help that Sigmund Freud, a neurologist, drew on myth
to analyze civilization and its discontents, and depended on

an unquantifiable process called talk therapy as a cure for the psychopathology of everyday life. Or that Auguste Comte, the father of modern sociology, promoted the establishment of a mystical secular project called the Religion of Humanity that would take the place of traditional (superstitious) religion. Or that economics—the social science that addresses the production, distribution, and consumption of goods and services—is famous for being the only field in which two people can get a Nobel Prize for expressing mutually contradictory ideas.[32]

Fast forward to 2004 and the founding of Facebook, the first web-based social utility capable of aggregating massive numbers of individuals and social groups into overlapping, concentric networks, and suddenly soft science starts speaking the same language as hard science. That language is Big Data.

In the ten-plus years since Facebook went live, everyone from retailers to medical researchers has been studying the behavior, patterns, and trends that arise out of people's online interactions with each other. Interestingly, data scientists, who separate the data wheat from the chaff and then feed "clean" data into scientific models to predict all kinds of human behavior, use the softest of terms—insight—to characterize their findings. Insight may not be as rock-solid as fact, but organizations are spending millions of dollars with companies such as PwC, Accenture, Palantir, SAS, and other consultancies to glean analytical insights from people's personal data. Indeed,

---

32   Dennis Alexis Valin Dittrich, Jokes About Economists and Economics, http://economicscience.net/content/JokEc.

the marriage of hard and soft science has given birth to a new discipline called "social physics." Alex Pentland, director of the MIT Connection Science and Human Dynamics Labs, coined the term to capture a new way of understanding human behavior through big data.[33]

It's official then: In everything from the sublime to the ridiculous, human beings influence each other. And we now have quantifiable data to prove it.

● ● ●

Public health researchers have learned two things from online social networks and from the pre-Internet Framingham Heart Study, a longitudinal cardiovascular study whose participants live in Framingham, Massachusetts:

A lot of human behavior is habitual.

Habitual behavior lends itself to mathematical modeling.

Both of these assertions rattle us. As Americans, we're inclined to reject claims that paint us individualists as herd followers. As it turns out, though, it doesn't take much to get us lone cowboys to behave like our neighbors. In a 2014 study investigating in-flight purchasing behavior, for example, a Stanford marketing researcher found that a passenger is approximately 30 percent more likely to buy a drink or a movie after witnessing his seatmate make a purchase.[34] If

---

33   Social Physics, http://socialphysics.media.mit.edu/about.

34   Pedro M. Gardete, "Social Effects in the In-Flight Marketplace: Characterization and Managerial Implications," 1.

we're susceptible to a stranger's influence—a stranger we may resent because he invades our personal space—how much more susceptible are we to the habits and recommendations of people we know and like?

Indeed, "emotional contagion"—the tendency to feel and express emotions similar to and influenced by those of others—only gathers momentum as it works its way through massive social networks.[35] Utilizing data from millions of Facebook users, social scientists Nicholas A. Christakis and James H. Fowler observed that rainfall not only influences the emotional content of a poster's status messages; it also affects the status messages of friends in other cities where it's not raining.[36] Much like a germ, a feeling in one place may spread to many parts of the globe on the same day and give rise to clusters of happy and unhappy individuals. The researchers conclude that the results of their study have significance for public well-being: "To the extent that clinical or policy maneuvers increase the happiness of one person, they may have cascade effects on others in their social networks, thereby enhancing the efficacy and cost-effectiveness of [an] intervention, and these results suggest that such cascade effects may be promoted online."[37]

---

35   Dictionary.com, "Emotional Contagion," http://dictionary.reference.com/browse/emotional-contagion.

36   Lorenzo Coviello, Yunkyu, Sohn, Adam D. I. Kramer, Cameron Marlow, Massimo Franceschetti, Nicholas A. Christakis, and James H. Fowler, "Detecting Emotional Contagion in Massive Social Networks," PLoS ONE 9, no. 3 (March 2014): abstract, http://journals.plos.org/plosone/article?id=10.1371/journal.pone.0090315.

37   Coviello et al., "Detecting Emotional Contagion in Massive Social Networks," 5.

A more controversial emotional contagion experiment by a core data science team at Facebook manipulated Facebook postings to emphasize either positive or negative content in an individual's News Feed (the continually updating list of posts, photos, videos, etc. in the middle of a personal home page).[38] The researchers wanted to see if "exposure to verbal affective expressions leads to similar verbal expressions, a form of emotional contagion."[39] They conducted two parallel experiments: In one, they reduced exposure to friends' positive emotional text; in the other, they reduced exposure to friends' negative emotional text.

As you might guess, people who saw more negative comments in their News Feed posted comparable negative comments; a more positive News Feed yielded more positive postings. In short, the results illustrate the phenomenon of emotional contagion in a vast social network.[40]

Arguably, Facebook's experiment, which manipulated users' emotions without their knowledge, was unethical.[41] (Facebook's

38   Facebook Help Center, "How Does News Feed Decide Which Stories to Show?" www.facebook.com/help/210346402339221.

39   Adam D. I. Kramer; Jamie E. Guillory, and Jeffrey T. Hancock "Experimental Evidence of Massive-Scale Emotional Contagion Through Social Networks," Proceedings of the National Academy of Sciences of the United States of America 111, no. 24 (June 2014), 1, http://www.pnas.org/content/111/24/8788.full.

40   Kramer et al., "Experimental Evidence of Massive-Scale Emotional Contagion Through Social Networks," 2.

41   Katy Waldman, "Facebook's Unethical Experiment," www.slate.com/articles/health_and_science/science/2014/06/facebook_unethical_experiment_it_made_news_feeds_happier_or_sadder_to_manipulate.html.

own justification for the experiment: users consent to this kind of manipulation when they agree to its terms of service.[42]) Facebook's tactics might give you pause, but the researchers drew an important implicit conclusion about managing chronic disease: "The well-documented connection between emotions and physical well-being suggests the importance of these findings for public health."[43]

Let's ask the question then: if the mere hint of a person's feeling about the weather or about a friend's emotional state can generate "synchrony," or simultaneous feeling, on a grand scale, what impact might our health habits have on people in our real-life and online social networks?

Judging by the growing body of research on "network interventions," our real-world and online social networks have a profound impact on what we eat, what kind of mood we're in, what drugs we take to stay healthy and how much we exercise.[44]

The World Health Organization has strict categories for communicable and noncommunicable (chronic) diseases, yet it appears to acknowledge that obesity—and malnutrition— are communicable epidemics that have spread globally. "Globesity," as the WHO calls the incidence of obesity around

42   Vindu Goel, "Facebook Tinkers With Users' Emotions in News Feed Experiment, Stirring Outcry," *New York Times*, www.nytimes.com/2014/06/30/technology/facebook-tinkers-with-users-emotions-in-news-feed-experiment-stirring-outcry.html.

43   Kramer et al., "Experimental Evidence of Massive-Scale Emotional Contagion Through Social Networks," 3.

44   Thomas W. Valente, "Network Interventions," Science 337, no. 6090 (2012), 49.

the world, contributes significantly to diabetes, cardiovascular disease, hypertension, stroke, and certain forms of cancer.[45] It also has the paradoxical effect of increasing body mass while exacerbating undernourishment. As with virtually all epidemics, globesity causes a range of problems, from an "increased risk of premature death to serious chronic conditions that reduce the overall quality of life."

Well-meaning US policy makers, who have witnessed a rise in adult obesity from 32 percent (2003–4) to 38 percent (2013–14), have worked to get calorie counts posted on food packages and restaurant menus.[46] They supported such measures in the belief that people will make healthier food choices if they know what they are eating. The results have been underwhelming: a Walmart healthier food initiative, for example, that mandated front-of-package labeling on certain products and offered price reductions as well, had little or no impact on shoppers' food purchases.[47] And a calorie labeling mandate in New York City restaurants, in place since 2008, has not led to a reduction in the calories of meals diners choose. The title of a *Health Affairs* research report points to the failure of the campaign: "Five Years

---

45   World Health Organization, "Controlling the Global Obesity Epidemic," www.who.int/nutrition/topics/obesity/en.

46   Aaron E. Carroll, "The Surprising Failure of Calorie Counts on Menus," *New York Times*, November 30, 2015, www.nytimes.com/2015/12/01/upshot/more-menus-have-calorie-labeling-but-obesity-rate-remains-high.html.

47   Carroll, "The Surprising Failure of Calorie Counts on Menus."

Later: Awareness Of New York City's Calorie Labels Declined, With No Changes In Calories Purchased."[48]

To confront the obesity epidemic, all too many policy makers lean on a legislative approach. The Obesity Action Coalition, for example, argues that people will buy fewer nonnecessity foods, such as sugary drinks, if these items are taxed a penny per ounce.[49] The dean of the Sanford School of Public Policy at Duke University has remarked as well that a rise in adult obesity could be thwarted by imposing a tax on soda.[50] These suggestions would be successful if *homo sapiens* had a rational approach to food. As nutritionists and marketing professors have observed, though, we eat for many different reasons, some of them emotional. We eat because we're happy. We eat because we're sad. Moreover, some psychologists and biologists (those soft and semisoft scientists) believe that for much of human history, we had a natural compulsion to eat fat-storing sugary foods. We're genetically coded to eat sugar over the course of a relatively short lifespan.

---

48   T. Jonathan Cantor, Alejandro Torres, Courtney Abrams, and Brian Elbel, "Five Years Later: Awareness Of New York City's Calorie Labels Declined, With No Changes in Calories Purchased," *Health Affairs*, November 2015, http://content.healthaffairs.org/content/34/11/1893. abstract.

49   Roberta R. Friedman, "A Soda Tax—Will It Change Anything," Obesity Action Coalition, http://www.obesityaction.org/educational-resources/resource-articles-2/nutrition/a-soda-tax-will-it-change-anything.

50   Sabrina Tavernise, "Obesity Rises Despite All Efforts to Fight It, U.S. Health Officials Say," *New York Times*, November 12, 2015, www.nytimes.com/2015/11/12/health/obesity-rises-despite-all-efforts-to-fight-it-us-health-officials-say.html.

"We didn't evolve as homo sapiens by eating healthy, because all we had to do was reproduce and survive until our mid-20's," says Dr. Leigh Gibson, a psychology professor at London's University of Roehampton.[51]

As with mood, social networks can also "transmit" obesity. Based on a Framingham Heart Study cohort (2007), data scientists Christakis and Fowler found that a person's chances of becoming obese "increased by 52 percent . . . if he or she had a friend who became obese in a given interval." Obesity rates increased too if a person's siblings or spouse were obese. Interestingly, physical proximity doesn't necessarily determine whether an individual will become obese. The researchers argue that the spread of obesity may depend less on "behavioral imitation" than on the "perception" that obesity in one's social circle is acceptable.[52]

So, post those calorie counts, restaurateurs! Tax away, legislators! But know that your rational approach to the obesity epidemic is likely to fail if you don't recognize the power of social networks to shape eating mores and values.

---

51   Julie Beck, "Our Moods, Our Foods," *The Atlantic,* March 6, 2014, www.theatlantic.com/health/archive/2014/03/our-moods-our-foods/284238.

52   Nicholas A. Christakis and James H. Fowler, "The Spread of Obesity in a Large Social Network Over 32 Years," *New England Journal of Medicine* 357 (July 26, 2007): 370–79, www.nejm.org/doi/full/10.1056/NEJMsa066082#t=article.

Nobody has understood the power of peer opinion better than the tobacco industry. Between the 1950s and 1971, TV advertisers made sure to put cigarettes in the hands of trusted newsmen (Ed Murrow), beloved cartoon characters (Fred Flintstone and Joe Camel), and ruggedly handsome cowboys (the Marlboro Man).[53] With the sophistication we've acquired over decades of hard-sell advertising, we can laugh off the tobacco industry's transparent efforts to associate cigarette smoking with freedom, authenticity, and independence, but by 1965, 43 percent of all American adults had taken the bait. The perception that only smart, attractive, and hip people smoked specific cigarette brands had bored through people's (pre-Internet) social networks like termites.

Fifty years' worth of warning labels on cigarette packages and restrictions on TV and radio advertising have helped reduce adult smoking rates to about 18 percent.[54] Even so, this current figure amounts to an estimated 42.1 million adult smokers. Some 480,000 of them die each year from smoking-related diseases—all preventable. These numbers pale when we compare them to the one billion people around the world who smoke, and the five million of them who die each year from tobacco-related illnesses.[55] The WHO dramatized these numbers with

---

53   "Tobacco," *Last Week Tonight With John Oliver*, www.youtube.com/watch?v=6UsHHOCH4q8.

54   Centers for Disease Control and Prevention, "Current Cigarette Smoking Among Adults in the United States," www.cdc.gov/tobacco/data_statistics/fact_sheets/adult_data/cig_smoking.

55   Sanjay Gupta, "Secondhand Smoke Kills 600,000 Worldwide Annually," http://thechart.blogs.cnn.com/2010/11/26/secondhand-

a sobering statistic regarding tobacco: one person dies every six seconds from cancer (lung and others), cardiovascular and metabolic diseases, respiratory diseases, and perinatal conditions (such as Sudden Infant Death Syndrome).[56]

In line with their research into large social networks, Christakis and Fowler examined how a smoking habit can spread from person to person. Once again they found that their Framingham Heart Study (1971–2003) participants were influenced by people in their network: When a spouse stopped smoking, a person's chances of smoking decreased by 67 percent. When a sibling stopped, the likelihood of smoking decreased by 25 percent. When a friend stopped, smoking could decrease by 36 percent. Coworkers in small firms could decrease a person's chances of smoking by 34 percent. And geographically close neighbors—people not necessarily within an individual's social network—had little or no effect at all.

In short, the old Mad Men advertisers understood what rational public health officials don't get: people will smoke—or not smoke—based on decisions undertaken by family, friends, and coworkers. And, as Christakis and Fowler learned, the more the merrier. A person is more apt to quit smoking if more than one person in his social network stops: "[W]hen a smoker runs

smoke-kills-600000-worldwide-annually.

56   Centers for Disease Control and Prevention, "Tobacco-Related Mortality," www.cdc.gov/tobacco/data_statistics/fact_sheets/health_effects/tobacco_related_mortality and Gupta, "Secondhand Smoke Kills 600,000."

out of easily available contacts with whom he or she can smoke, he or she may be more likely to quit."[57]

Christakis, Fowler, and their colleagues also studied the transmission of heavy alcohol habits in an offspring cohort of the Framingham Heart Study, that is, predominantly second generation (1971) Framingham study participants. Their findings echo the results of the obesity and tobacco studies: "Alcohol consumption behavior among individuals and others in their social networks is highly correlated."[58] People were 50 percent more likely to abuse alcohol if the person they were directly connected to drank heavily. They were 36 percent more likely to overdo it if a friend of a friend drank heavily and 15 percent more likely if influenced by a friend of a friend of a friend. At four degrees of separation, the social network contagion just about disappears—as in studies concerning obesity, smoking, happiness, depression, and loneliness.[59]

Even abstainers can be enticed into acquiring an unhealthy drinking habit. The Framingham researchers speculate that the popular image of women as moderate drinkers actually provoked greater alcohol abuse among women in social networks.

• ◆ •

---

57   Nicholas A. Christakis and James H. Fowler, "The Collective Dynamics of Smoking in a Large Social Network," *New England Journal of Medicine* 358 (2008): 2256–57.

58   J. Niels Rosenquist, Joanne Murabito, James H. Fowler, and Nicholas A. Christakis, "The Spread of Alcohol Consumption Behavior in a Large Social Network," *Annals of Internal Medicine* 152 (April 6, 2010), 6.

59   Rosenquist et al., "The Spread of Alcohol Consumption Behavior," 5.

While people tend to abuse food, tobacco and alcohol if they model themselves on likeminded family and friends, social networks also have the potential to help people adopt healthier behaviors. Indeed, Alex Pentland's work at MIT suggests that modifying the "social fabric" can help individuals change their behavior much more effectively than if they are offered personal incentives. In one experiment, Pentland and his associates rewarded buddies. If a person became more physically active, the reward went to the encouraging buddy. "What happens is everybody's looking at everybody and saying, 'Are you being active?'" Pentland says. "Even when we ran out of monetary incentives, people stuck with their higher level of physical activity during the period of observation. What we did is change the social fabric. We made being active a topic of conversation, a topic of social pressure, of prestige, of interest."[60]

Christakis and Fowler have reached the same conclusion about social networks that offer peer support for people struggling to lose weight, quit smoking, and stop drinking to excess: "Network phenomena might be exploited to spread positive health behaviors, in part because people's perceptions of their own risk of illness may depend on the people around them." As they assert throughout all their research studies, "Since people are connected, their health is also connected."[61]

---

60   Sandy Pentland, "Social Physics: How Good Ideas Spread," Google Talk, https://www.youtube.com/watch?v=HMBl0ttu-Ow.

61   Christakis and Fowler, "The Spread of Obesity in a Large Social Network," 378.

Indeed, research on emotional contagion shows that social networks can behave in positive ways. Let's look at the challenge of getting cardiac patients to take a recommended aspirin every day. Longitudinal data from 2,724 members of the Framingham Heart Study (2012) reveals that an individual is more likely to take that aspirin if his friends take it too. Men are more likely to take aspirin if a brother or male friend takes it; women are more likely to take aspirin if a brother or female friend takes it.[62] While no one single person can influence absolutely everybody else in her social network, the study researchers nonetheless observed that "[p]harmacotherapy is a behavior, and so we should not be surprised by the fact that people's drug-taking behavior is related to the behavior of those around them, and to the events occurring in those around them."[63]

The aspirin study highlights the role social networks can play in helping patients self-manage chronic disease. A comparable British study about diabetics (2014) found that "being connected to voluntary and community groups was related to key dimensions of self-monitoring and skill and technique acquisition . . . as well as to better physical health and emotional well-being." The researchers found that a supportive social network is even more effective in keeping diabetics "engaged and active in normal life" than family members: "[P]

62   Kate W. Strully, James H. Fowler, Joanne M. Murabio, Emelia J. Benjamin, Daniel Levy, Nicholas A. Christakis, "Aspirin Use and Cardiovascular Events in Social Networks," Social Science and Medicine 74 (2012): abstract, http://fowler.ucsd.edu/aspirin_use_and_cardiovascular_events_in_social_networks.pdf.

63   Strully et al., "Aspirin Use and Cardiovascular Events," 1129.

eople with poorer health or less healthy behaviours tended to have more children living nearby."[64] In effect, medical care and patient adherence constitute only one part of diabetes disease management. Helpful activities by those who are not healthcare providers—friends, partners and "weak tie" network relationships—also contribute to positive health outcomes.

Notably, patients with no links to community groups showed a decline in healthy behaviours.[65]

The British researchers also found that healthcare costs for diabetic patients who received emotional and practical support from their social network were generally one-half the cost for patients who didn't have this kind of support, largely because patients with network ties could avoid long hospital stays.[66]

One last example of the beneficial "contagious" effects of a social network: The Palo Alto Medical Foundation (PAMF) combined big data analytics and social networking to design LinkAges, a community-based mutual aid program aimed at combating loneliness among the elderly. The program is much more than a nice-to-have. Older people who say they are lonely have a 45 percent greater risk of dying and a 60 percent greater risk of experiencing problems with walking, climbing stairs,

---

64   David Reeves, Christian Blickem, Ivaylo Vassilev, Helen Brooks, Anne Kennedy, Gerry Richardson, and Anne Rogers, "The Contribution of Social Networks to the Health and Self-Management of Patients with Long-Term Conditions: A Longitudinal Study," PLoS ONE, June 2014, 8, http://journals.plos.org/plosone/article?id=10.1371/journal.pone.0098340.

65   Reeves et al., "The Contribution of Social Networks," 8.

66   Reeves et al., "The Contribution of Social Networks," 10.

lifting, and other everyday activities.[67] Overseen by internist and chief innovation and technology officer Paul Tang, LinkAges provides a service-exchange network. When participants trade skills and services, they earn hours in a "time bank" that they can use when they need a ride to the airport, a cooking lesson, a computer demonstration, etc. The Commonwealth Fund observes that LinkAges creates a sense of group cohesion based on a neighborly pay-it-forward plan, not on a self-interested I'll-scratch-your-back-if-you-scratch-mine system. In keeping with Alex Pentland's notion of social physics, personal acts of altruism sustain the entire social fabric, not simply individuals who obligate themselves to do and receive favors.

A Commonwealth Fund report underscores what makes LinkAges indispensable for managing chronic disease. An older female patient missed three follow-up breast cancer appointments at PAMF. An interviewer for a PAMF ethnographic study learned that the patient couldn't afford the seventy-five dollar taxi ride from her home. The patient was able to overcome this particular hurdle by joining LinkAges. As Tang observes, "The ways in which seemingly nonmedical information about a patient affects her healthcare, I think, are a really big part of the gap between where we are and where we need to be in managing diseases."[68]

---

67   Susan L. Hayes, Douglas McCarthy, and Sarah Klein, "linkAges: Building Support Systems for Seniors Living Independently in the Community," September 2015, www.commonwealthfund.org/-/ media/files/publications/innovation-profile/2015/sep/1835_hayes_ linkages_v2.pdf.

68   Hayes et al., "linkAges: Building Support Systems for Seniors Living Independently in the Community."

By now you see that the power of social networks, when properly harnessed, can help patients manage their chronic conditions. That's why we constructed a social network at Ochsner to help patients with congestive heart failure control their salt intake. The system isn't even complicated. We find out who prepares and/or shops for a patient's food. Then we ask that person to watch a short educational video about low-sodium diets. That's it. And we accomplished two things: We've gotten information about low sodium to the right person. And we've activated the patient's social network—which foments connections on other health-related matters as well. The net result of their involvement and secondary education reduced the chance of the patient being rehospitalized by 42 percent. Ultimately, the social network makes it possible for any person to have a positive impact on another individual's life.

Your mother was right when she said you are the company you keep. Who better than she knew that the most important question for her family and her community was, "How do we get people to make good decisions and follow through on them?"

Turns out that's the same question data scientists, social scientists, and public health experts ask about how to get people to make good decisions about their health.

In the real and digital worlds, people transmit and receive emotions and habits via the company they keep. The mission for healthcare policy makers is to turn the madness of the crowd—when people copy bad health habits from their friends, family, and coworkers—to the wisdom of the crowd—when people adopt life-enhancing health habits and stick to them.

That's never been an easy task, but the hard and soft scientists are showing us through their analysis of social network data how to get started.

CHAPTER 3

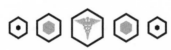

What Healthcare Can Learn from Las Vegas and Madison Avenue

Admit it. Every now and then, you buy a Powerball ticket. Why not? If you win, the payout is enormous. Of course the odds are about 1 in 292 million that you will actually win, but it only costs two dollars to play, and you have to pay to win. And in the highly unlikely event that you do win—nothing in your life will ever be the same again.

If only people could feel the same thrill about eating right and exercising—two activities, realistically speaking, that would help Americans reduce the probability of getting diabetes, high blood pressure, and congestive heart failure.

As it turns out, the creative minds behind Powerball and other games of chance rely on behavioral research that examines what motivates people to invest in an activity that promises so little yet keeps them coming back for more. Indeed, casinos are masterful at engineering environments that lift you out of your everyday life into a leisure wonderland of blackjack tables, restaurants, shopping, indoor auto races, and ventriloquist stage shows. The casino is designed to deliver a Monte Carlo experience that people look forward to repeating again and again.

In our more reflective moments, we see that the mind games casinos subject us to are transparent, if not downright devious: Eliminate clocks and windows so players lose track of time. Use chips instead of real money at the tables so our losses don't feel so bad. When someone wins at slots, be sure there's lots of noise and celebration so that we all believe we can win too. Considering that casinos are so good at manipulating us to spin the wheel one more time, the healthcare industry would do well to learn from these tactics with the more noble goal of promoting healthy, sustainable, and economically feasible lifestyle habits.

• ⬢ •

The gaming industry has known for decades what behavioral psychologist B. F. Skinner recognized in the mid-1970s: "All gambling systems are based on variable-ratio schedules of reinforcement, although their effects are usually attributed to feelings."[69] In common parlance, Skinner believed that gambling consists of an intentional action (betting that two playing cards will add up to twenty-one); a consequence (winning), and continued repetition of that action in the unproven hope that the consequence will be good again.[70] Skinner used this gambling sequence to make a larger point about human behavior, namely, that an "important factor contributing to the probability that an individual will turn over money, either for other money or for goods, is the schedule on which he is reinforced for doing so."[71]

Hitting a tennis ball against a wall over and over again might demonstrate Skinner's reinforcement schedule more simply: You swing the racquet, the ball hits the wall, it comes back at you a second or so later, and you keep swinging until you finally miss the ball. You begin again because the activity is rewarding and suspenseful.

Skinner also believed that with increasingly sophisticated technology, scientists would be able to link variable scheduling behavior to the body's physiological responses. His goal: take the guesswork out of analyzing human behavior.

---

69   Reza Habib and Mark R. Dixon, "Neurobehavioral Evidence for the 'Near-Miss' Effect in Pathological Gamblers," *Journal of the Experimental Analysis of Behavior* 93, no. 3 (2010): 313–28, www.ncbi. nlm.nih.gov/pmc/articles/PMC2861872.

70   Terry J. Knapp, "Behaviorism and Public Policy: B. F. Skinner's Views on Gambling," *Behavioral and Social Issues* 7, no. 2 (1997): 129–39, http://journals.uic.edu/ojs/index.php/bsi/article/viewFile/311/2939.

71   Knapp, "Behaviorism and Public Policy," 132.

A new generation of behaviorists has built on Skinner's "VR schedules" by studying a range of factors that appear to encourage pathological gambling. Psychologists Jeffrey N. Weatherly and Mark R. Dixon suggest that pathological gambling may involve a "dynamic interaction between programmed contingencies, verbal behavior, and various contextual stimuli (i.e., financial status, race, comorbid psychological disorders)." That is, psychological and social realities can exacerbate extreme gambling tendencies. Edmund Fantino and Stephanie Stolarz-Fantino contributed the delay reduction hypothesis to behavioral science: People are averse to delays, and when a reward—imagined or real—is in sight, they will repeat an action in the hope of attaining a positive outcome. Near misses, frequent in games of chance, stimulate repeated behaviors. Pathological gamblers believe that a near miss in one gambling instance could lead to a win in the next. So, try, try again.

Advertisers and market researchers have benefited from gambling studies. After all, Pepsico, Coca-Cola and Tyson Foods, to name a few, did not make the *Fortune 500* list because they sell you a one-off bag of potato chips or an occasional jar of tomato sauce.[72] Food scientist and market researcher Howard Moskowitz admits as much when he talks about the "bliss point," the "sensory profile where you like food the most."[73] Moskowitz describes this sensory profile as a parabola: As you

---

72 *Fortune 500* List, http://fortune.com/fortune500.

73 Howard Moskowitz, "The Bliss Point," *The New York Times* | Retro Report Voices, www.retroreport.org/voices/the-bliss-point/.

increase the amount of sugar in a product, liking goes up, peaks, reaches a bliss point and goes down. Because the bliss point is different for each person, Moskowitz has helped the food industry create various product lines by playing around with key ingredients, notably sugar, salt, and fat. Does the bliss point make food addictive? Absolutely not, Moskowitz says. "It just makes it delicious."

Almost without a doubt, Skinner and his successors would take issue with Howard Moskowitz. Not only does that potato chip trigger the desire for another chip ("Nobody can eat just one"), but that desire is observable with technology. One positron emission tomography (PET) study, for example, compared the amount of dopamine in a normal brain with the brains of food and cocaine abusers. The PET scans showed that food and drug addicts both have fewer than average dopamine receptors. The result: weaker dopamine signals are sent between cells—and addicts need more drug or more food to feel high, satiated, etc.[74] Sugar appears to have the same effect on the brain as smoking, alcohol, and cocaine. Indeed, researchers at Connecticut College found that laboratory rats spent as much time eating Oreos—cookies rich in sugar and fat—as getting high on cocaine or morphine. The Oreo-eating rats were also tested for a protein called c-Fos, a known marker of neural activity in the region of brain that controls the feeling of pleasure. Oreos beat out both drugs by a "significant margin."[75]

---

74   Tom McKay, "What Happens to Your Brain on Sugar, Explained by Science," Science.Mic, http://mic.com/articles/88015/what-happens-to-your-brain-on-sugar-explained-by-science#.HFKDRfxa5.

75   McKay, "What Happens to Your Brain on Sugar."

The pleasure-inducing properties of Oreos and other snacks "may explain why some people can't resist these foods despite the fact that they know they are bad for them," says Joseph Schroeder, director of the behavioral neuroscience program at Connecticut College.

It's safe to say that food manufacture—like casino gambling—is specifically designed to influence our eating behavior.

Insights into the physiological and behavioral response to food are enormously valuable to food marketers.

A Federal Trade Commission (FTC) study reported that the US food industry spent $1.79 billion marketing food to youth in 2006. Some $1.29 billion of that went toward marketing fast-food restaurant foods, carbonated beverages, and breakfast cereals.[76] The healthcare industry might envy how well food marketers understand their audience. First, marketing executives create advertising campaigns aimed at market "segments." What appeals to a two-year-old won't appeal to a seventeen-year-old. Second, no venue is ignored. Food marketers routinely partner with schools, where they spent nearly $150 million (2009) on promoting carbonated and noncarbonated drinks. And as eyeballs have moved from television to mobile devices,

---

76 Federal Trade Commission, "A Review of Food Marketing to Children and Adolescents: Follow-Up Report," 2012, https://www.ftc.gov/sites/default/files/documents/reports/review-food-marketing-children-and-adolescents-follow-report/121221foodmarketingreport.pdf. This was a follow-up to the 2008 report.

food companies are moving their marketing dollars from TV advertising to new-media outlets—$122.5 million in 2009.[77]

Not only do food marketers take advantage of the bliss point in the products themselves. They also play on what children love: popular movies, TV programs, cartoon characters, toys, websites, video games, and theme parks. *Ice Age: Dawn of the Dinosaurs*, the *Madagascar* movies, and *Night at the Museum* were prominent in 2009 and were used to promote a wide array of sugary products, according to the FTC report.

Arguably, marketing to adults in the Internet era is even easier than marketing to children, because adults voluntarily offer up so much information about themselves on Facebook, Pinterest, Instagram and other social media websites. Predictive analytics, a branch of data mining that analyzes consumers' personal and shopping habits in order to project future buying habits, has become an essential part of the retail toolkit. Target, for example, famously used shopper data to learn that people change their shopping patterns and brand loyalties when they are about to become new parents. The company ascertained that it had to reach the new mom in her second trimester, when expectant mothers begin buying vitamins, maternity clothes, and other pregnancy-related items. Once Target gets expectant mothers and fathers hooked, the store can turn them into much-desired repeat customers.

"As soon as we get them buying diapers from us, they're going to start buying everything else too," Target statistician

---

77   Federal Trade Commission, "A Review of Food Marketing to Children and Adolescents."

Andrew Pole told *The New York Times* in 2012. "If you're rushing through the store, looking for bottles, and you pass orange juice, you'll grab a carton. Oh, and there's that new DVD I want. Soon, you'll be buying cereal and paper towels from us, *and keep coming back*."[78]

Through uniquely assigned customer ID numbers, Target compiles a head-spinning amount of data on how customers interact with the store: Did they use a credit card or coupon to make a purchase? Did they fill out a survey, mail in a refund, call the customer service line, open a store email, visit the Target website? Thanks to the lists Target buys or information it gleans from your Facebook page—your age, marital status, address, salary, magazine subscriptions, pharmacy prescriptions, reading habits, charitable donations, and political leanings, to name a few—the big box retailer has become a leader in the science of "habit formation." In short, it turns bits of stray information into data it can mine for insights into buyer behavior and consumption trends.

If Powerball, Caesar's Palace, and Target can use our personal data to entice us to gamble and shop, why shouldn't healthcare organizations use it to entice us into healthier lifestyle habits?

Habit formation research shows that, to some extent, they can.

In 2015, a team of British public health researchers worked with a cohort of adults fifty and older to study what effect a

---

78   Italics mine. Charles Duhigg, "How Companies Learn Your Secrets," *New York Times,* Feb. 12, 2012, www.nytimes.com/2012/02/19/ magazine/shopping-habits.html.

change in one partner's health behavior had on the other partner. Among 3,722 participating adults, men and women were more likely to change their health behavior for the better if their partner changed too. That is, witnessing a partner make a change had greater impact than simply living with somebody who entered the relationship with good health habits.[79]

Of course, smokers who had a consistently healthy, nonsmoking partner had significantly higher odds of quitting smoking, and inactive individuals had higher odds of becoming physically active if their partner engaged in regular exercise. But smokers and physically inactive people had *even greater odds* of taking on healthy habits if they actually saw their partner stop smoking or start exercising.

Eating habits were a different matter. Overweight individuals were not especially influenced by partners who entered into the relationship with a normal body mass index (BMI)—but *seeing* an overweight partner lose weight was associated with three times higher odds of weight loss.

The British researchers wanted to know why having a partner who becomes healthy is more persuasive than a partner

79 S. E. Jackson, A. Steptoe, and J. Wardle, "The Influence of Partner's Behavior on Health Behavior Change: The English Longitudinal Study of Ageing," *JAMA Internal Medicine* 175, no. 3 (2015), www.psychologie.uzh.ch/studium/master/abschluss/artikel/Artikel_Scholz--SOB--HS15___2015-10-01.pdf. See also Melissa M. Franks, Cleveland G. Shields, Eunjung Lim, Laura P. Sands, Stacey Mobley, and Carol J. Boushey, "I Will If You Will: Similarity in Married Partners' Readiness to Change Health Risk Behaviors," *Health Education and Behavior*, April 15, 2011, http://heb.sagepub.com/content/early/2011/04/13/1090198111402824.abstract.

who is consistently healthy. They point to a US study aptly titled "I Will If You Will: Similarity in Married Partners' Readiness to Change Health Risk Behaviors." It suggests that "people feel more able to change their behavior if their partner is also motivated to change." The American researchers argue too that "successful behavior change in one partner may encourage the other to try to change their behavior." This is the case whether one partner initiates the change and the other follows suit or if both partners simultaneously decide to become more healthy.

Alas, losing weight, exercising, or giving up tobacco is not as simple as watching a partner get healthy, as a team of researchers at the University of Birmingham (U.K.) discovered. In 2012, they published the results of a "social modeling" experiment designed to "examine whether observing someone else making either predominantly 'unhealthy' or 'healthy' eating choices at a buffet would influence food choice."

The researchers hypothesized that a "young female" participant who observed another young female choose unhealthy foods (cookies, etc.) would herself choose unhealthy foods. Likewise, a young female who observed another participant choose healthy foods (carrots, etc.) would choose healthy foods. The actual results, however, did not fully match researchers' expectations.

The researchers found that participants who saw another person choosing healthy foods did not significantly choose more healthy foods. They ultimately had to question whether healthier food choices "can be encouraged as a result of modelling."

And yet other food choice experiments have yielded precisely opposite conclusions, as the Birmingham researchers acknowledge. In 2008, pediatric researchers at SUNY-Buffalo found that "overweight children ate substantially more when alone than when in the presence of a peer." Moreover, children were also more likely to consume healthy snacks if another child consumed them too.[80] A 2009 Dutch-Canadian study observed that young women ate more vegetables when exposed to a peer eating a large number of vegetables, and fewer vegetables when exposed to a peer eating a small number of vegetables (or to a peer eating no vegetables at all).[81] And a 1980 study of preschoolers at the University of Illinois (Urbana-Champaign) showed that very young children can be influenced to choose healthier foods if they are seated next to children who prefer healthier options—even when those young children have stated a preference for unhealthy foods.[82] The Birmingham researchers offered up the possibility of design flaws in their experiment because they could not reproduce the results of these previous studies. They also wondered if food choices are simply "less

---

80   Sarah-Jeanne Salvy, Elizabeth Kieffer, and Leonard H. Epstein, "Effects of Social Context on Overweight and Normal-Weight Children's Food Selection," *Eating Behavior* 9, no. 2 (2008): 190–96, http://www.ncbi.nlm.nih.gov/pmc/articles/PMC2365747.

81   Roel C. J. Hermans, Junilla K. Larsen, C. Peter Herman, and Rutger C. M. E. Engels, "Effects of Social Modeling on Young Women's Nutrient-Dense Food Intake," *Appetite* 53, no. 1 (2009): 135–38, www.sciencedirect.com/science/article/pii/S0195666309005005.

82   Leann Lipps Birch, "Effects of Peer Models' Food Choices and Eating Behaviors on Preschoolers' Food Preferences," *Child Development* 51, no. 2 (1980): 489–96.

susceptible to social modelling . . . because people feel sure of their food likes and dislikes and do not need to look to others to guide these preferences."[83]

• ⬡ •

The goal of these various habit formation studies is to see what makes human behavior "normative" in controlled experiments—and then use the findings to shape behavior in the casino, the retail store, or the food court. Increasingly, behavioral studies rely on data gathered from relatively large cohorts consisting of hundreds, thousands, and even millions of participants. The larger the study group, the more legitimately researchers can conclude that, given specific actions, influences, and rewards, most of us will respond the way our friends, family, and neighbors do to a range of issues.

A case in point: One 2008 investigation set out to determine if 810 Californians could be influenced to conserve energy simply by being informed that their fellow Californians were already conserving energy.[84] Indeed, previous research (by

83   Eric Robinson and Suzanne Higgs, "Food Choices in the Presence of 'Healthy' and "Unhealthy' Eating Partners," *British Journal of Nutrition* 109, no. 4 (2013): 1–7, http://pure-oai.bham.ac.uk/ws/files/17764865/Robinson_Food_Choices_British_Journal_Nutrition_2013.pdf.

84   Jessica M. Nolan, P. Wesley Schultz, Robert B. Cialdini, Noah J. Goldstein, and Vladas Griskevicius, "Normative Social Influence is Underdetected," *Personality and Social Psychology Bulletin* 34, no. 7 (2008): 913-23, http://citeseerx.ist.psu.edu/viewdoc/download?doi=10.1.1.431.5682&rep=rep1&type=pdf.

one of the study designers) found that households receiving "normative information describing the amount recycled by an average neighborhood family increased both the amount and frequency of their subsequent curbside recycling behaviors." This social "priming," or subtle, imperceptible persuasion, "can produce strong and perceptible changes in behavior," as it did in the energy conservation study: Even though participants believed their neighbors' conservation habits had little or no impact on their own habits, "results showed that the descriptive norm"—that neighbors recycled their plastics, papers and glass—actually had the strongest effect on participants' energy conservation behaviors. That is, normative information spurred people to conserve more energy than any of the standard appeals that are often used to stimulate energy conservation, such as protecting the environment, being socially responsible, or even saving money."

Perhaps most interesting of all was that the descriptive norm—that neighbors practiced recycling—had a "powerful but underdetected "effect on a desirable social behavior.

Further, the researchers believe that if the study participants suspected that their neighbors' conservation habits were influencing them to change their own conservation habits, the study participants would not have done as much recycling.

It's sobering to think how easily we are influenced by neighbors we may not even know, and how unaware we are of their influence over us. The researchers concluded that "appealing to people to do the right thing, or to protect the environment, rarely succeeds in increasing levels of pro-environmental behavior." Merely letting people know what other people around them are doing turns out to be the most effective motivator for "doing the right thing."

Of course the human inclination to copy their neighbors' actions does not always lead to socially desirable results. A 2011 study involving 80,000 participants found that media depictions of risk-taking behavior increased participants' own risk-taking actions. It didn't matter what kind of research methods the study authors used (experimental, correlational, longitudinal), what kind of media they showed (video games, movies, advertising, TV, music), or what risk-related outcomes they measured (smoking, drinking, risky driving, sexual behavior): exposure to risk-glorifying media content increased participants' risk-taking "behaviors, cognitions, and emotions" in the real world.[85]

Indeed, the same researchers who designed the California conservation study found that some normative descriptions can produce "unintended and undesirable boomerang effects."[86] For example, a college campaign targeting alcohol consumption might motivate students who previously consumed less alcohol than the norm to consume more. The study authors had to

---

85 Peter Fischer, Tobias Greitemeyer, Andreas Kastenmüller, Claudia Vogrincic , and Anne Sauer, "The Effects of Risk-Glorifying Media Exposure on Risk-Positive Cognitions, Emotions, and Behaviors: A Meta-Analytic Review," *Psychology Bulletin* 137, no. 3 (2011): 367-90,http://uncw.edu/commonreading/documents/EffectsofRisk-GlorifyingMedia.pdf.

86 P. Wesley Schultz, Jessica M. Nolan, Robert B. Cialdini, Noah J. Goldstein, and Vladas Griskevicius, "The Constructive, Destructive, and Reconstructive Power of Social Norms," *Psychological Science* 18, no. 5 (2007): 429–34, https://jsmf.org/meetings/2008/july/social%20 norms%20Cialdini.pdf.

conclude that "although providing descriptive normative information may decrease an undesirable behavior among individuals who perform that behavior at a rate above the norm, the same message may actually serve to increase the undesirable behavior among individuals who perform that behavior at a rate below the norm."

Even here students may be reinfluenced to believe that the majority of their peers think binge drinking is "lame." Communicating an "injunctive norm"—a social behavior that serves as a de facto law (such as speaking quietly in the library or yielding the right-of-way on escalators)—may actually influence them to maintain their lower-than-typical college drinking habits.[87]

In short, so much of the behavior we engage in is the result of imitation. Moreover, we conform, unwittingly, to the habits and values of the people around us, even when we insist we march to a different drummer.

B. F. Skinner, who understood that people could be induced to engage in and repeat certain behaviors under specifically designed circumstances, disliked state lotteries because they claimed people were "free to buy or not to buy tickets," when, in fact, physiological and behavioral imperatives overrode personal volition. "Gambling is wrong," Skinner wrote, "not because it ruins some people or is tabooed by a church, but

---

87   Schultz et al., "The Constructive, Destructive, and Reconstructive Power of Social Norms."

because it commits a person to repetitious, stultifying behavior" they cannot subdue.[88]

Healthcare providers and policy makers need to recognize that casinos and retail stores have been brilliant at turning occasional patrons into repeat customers. And these big-box enterprises have accomplished their goal largely by understanding how human beings are inclined *by nature* to behave in a casino, at the mall, on an airplane, on a college campus. The scientists and marketers who study habit formation are mining big data samples to do the very thing that can help reduce chronic disease: identify unhealthy behaviors and trends and then design psychologically clever programs to do what you want people to do, namely, change their health habits for the better. The science behind habit formation and behavior change exists—and it's not valuable only to the marketers at Caesar's and Target. Isn't it time for the healthcare industry to put the strategies of the gaming table to good use in doctors' offices, healthcare centers, and communities?

---

88   Knapp, "Behaviorism and Public Policy."

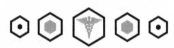

CHAPTER 4

Why Going to the Doctor Might Be the Least Effective Way to Get Well

Whenever we're under the weather, injured, or facing a more serious health issue, our immediate thought is to go to the doctor. The doctor will know what is wrong and will be able to provide the medication or treatment necessary to achieve an optimal level of health—right?

Well, we're finding more and more that this isn't always the case. In fact, going to the doctor might be the least effective way to get well. I'll show you what I mean by sharing a story about my mother-in-law and her physician.

My mother-in-law is seventy-nine years old and lives in a wealthy retirement community in Florida. She works out three times a week and is perfectly healthy. In fact, I'm sure that she'll outlive me.

One day, my healthy mother-in-law went to her general practitioner for a check-up. For some reason, he decided to order an ECG on this particular day. We're not sure why the test was ordered because my mother-in-law wasn't displaying any symptoms. Nevertheless, the results of the ECG showed an abnormality, which is not unusual given the fact that she's seventy-nine years old.

The abnormality itself was an extremely common condition and not one that generally serves as a cause for concern. I know this because I had my mother-in-law fax her ECG results to me and I saw that the abnormality was a benign premature ventricular contraction (PVC).

Though a benign PVC is something that most of us would display in an ECG at some point, my mother-in-law's physician expressed serious concerns about her cardiovascular health and advised her to see a cardiologist at once.

I, on the other hand, advised my mother-in-law not to go to a cardiologist because I knew that it would only result in more unnecessary tests. Her physician certainly should have known that the PVC didn't necessitate a cardiologist. Nevertheless, because she's seventy-nine years old and can afford it, he insisted that she visit the specialist. The language he used to describe the condition and his urgent recommendation completely terrified my mother-in-law, and she rushed in to see the cardiologist.

The cardiologist then ordered a computed tomography angiography (CTA), which is an expensive and unnecessary test. This created undue stress on her body, not to mention a spike in her anxiety. As expected, the CTA results showed some blockages in her heart arteries. What the cardiologist didn't share with her is that, taking her age into account, the blockages are common and not cause for alarm or further treatment because of her lack of symptoms. Instead, his office informed my healthy mother-in-law that she was in need of an emergency coronary angiogram.

At that point I advised her not to undergo the angiogram and to see me instead. She flew from Florida to New Orleans, and I had a test done on her that can only be done in four or five places in the country. I wasn't surprised to find that the results showed a noncritical blockage, which her body was bypassing naturally. These results allowed me to finally succeed in convincing my mother-in-law that the abnormality the initial ECG and other tests found was not a big deal and that none of the recommended testing had been necessary. When she returned home and explained the situation to her doctor, he sent her a certified letter firing her from his practice.

I believe he overreacted, not only to her decision to seek my medical advice, but initially in his recommendations for further treatment. This was not a situation of a misdiagnosis on her doctor's part, but an error in judgment.

Perhaps the doctor was inexperienced or misinformed, so he didn't realize that he was overreacting and potentially exposing her to injury or complications. Ironically, he seemed to believe that he was doing the right thing for my mother-in-law, and that I was interfering with the quality of care he was providing.

Unfortunately, my mother-in-law's story is not a singular case. What's worse is that if this story had been about a woman whose son-in-law wasn't a cardiologist, it's likely that she would have rushed in for an emergency intervention she didn't need. The cardiologist would then have put a stent in her heart artery and hopefully, at seventy-nine years old, she wouldn't suffer a complication from the procedure itself.

The woman and her insurance company would have spent thousands of dollars. She would be sore following the procedure and possibly experience bleeding. After a few days in the hospital, she would be sent home with blood-thinning medication, which would then cause her to bruise all the time. At the end of it all, her health would be a fraction of what it was prior to the unnecessary procedure and testing. Interestingly, the woman would believe that the doctor actually saved her life.

The dichotomy lies between our culture and the system. Doctors are usually thought of as experts who have information that the patients themselves cannot comprehend. This creates a culture of patients going to physicians and not questioning the information they receive, rarely obtaining second or third opinions, and then being subjected to tests, medications, and procedures that are not necessary and perhaps even dangerous.

Many procedures and medications do save lives and are absolutely necessary, and so the issues are complex and lay within the system. The first issue is what was discussed in earlier chapters: physicians often aren't given enough time to understand a patient's health, history, and lifestyle, as well as other factors, such as depression, work and home circumstances, exposure to secondhand smoke, and so on.

The expectations of documentation, liability testing, mandated recordkeeping, and more, further burden physicians and distract them from providing quality care through thorough conversation and examination.

This issue leads into the next: as healthcare practitioners, we are overprescribing.

Forced to rush through patient visits, physicians often provide a prescription for a pill and move on to the next appointment. This isn't solely due to the physician's time constraints, but dates back to yet more issues within the system. Economic factors also come into play here. A physician cannot risk being sued for a misdiagnosis, or even a missed diagnosis, as was the case with my mother-in-law. Fear and obligation drive physicians to order tests that don't necessarily serve a purpose. This actually contributes to the extremely high healthcare costs in the United States. Not to mention the avoidable anxiety and anguish that people go through because they place so much trust in their doctors. Most of the time, prescribing a pill is the most a doctor can actually do, and it is often what is expected by the patient.

Take the case of antibiotics. The Centers for Disease Control (CDC) tell us that anywhere from one-third to one-half of the antibiotics prescribed annually are unnecessary, because the cause of the illness is viral, not bacterial. The result is not only harm and costs to patients (antibiotics are a leading cause of adverse events from drugs), but, even worse, antibiotic-resistant bacteria such as methicillin-resistant Staphylococcus aureus (MRSA). Each year, antibiotic-resistant bacteria cause more than 2 million illnesses and 23,000 deaths. Recently however, programs are being built, such as the one at Ochsner, that provide feedback to physicians about their individual antibiotic prescribing coupled with resource guides for patients about alternatives. These real-time reports have been shown to dramatically reduce the frequency of inappropriate antibiotic prescribing.

To yet further complicate the issue of medication safety, most drugs are tested on patients who are twenty-one to sixty-five years of age, then released for patients of any age. This can become problematic since we don't know how older patients will react to certain medications.

As you know, anything you put in your system that can help you, can also hurt you, and sometimes at the same time. One of the unfortunate things about aging is that the dose that would produce a small amount of toxicity in a younger person now may produce a higher amount of toxicity in the older person. Therefore, drugs that have been shown to be of value for people in their forties might prove toxic for people in their seventies.

Unfortunately, some physicians may not consider these factors when prescribing medications to older patients; it often takes a trained geriatrician or a clinical pharmacist. It's important to note that this does not touch upon the issue of drug interactions, a significant problem that often takes a clinical pharmacologist to recognize.

So what's the good news?

In light of this information, we initiated a clinic in my institution, Ochsner–SafeMed, where clinical pharmacologists evaluate elderly patients and their prescriptions in order to determine which medications are necessary and which can be discontinued. As a result, people are taken off drugs that their bodies don't need, and their quality of life actually improves.

This is an example of a solution to an identified issue, and such clinics are opening up throughout the country, attempting to resolve various issues within our current medical system.

Though it may not always seem like it, we are actually moving toward a system that pays for the quality of care provided, not for the procedures performed. Medicine is going in the right direction because we have moved toward holding doctors accountable for outcomes, not just for showing up and prescribing something. *Doctors now have to demonstrate that they create desirable outcomes, including quality of life, survival, and other measurable results.* This change in the payment model has been called moving "from volume to value" and will ultimately benefit patients.

Another example of such progress can been seen through the fact that medical doctors are now required to take the board exams every ten years. While this helps to ensure that practitioners are maintaining up-to-date practices, medical errors are the third leading cause of death in the United States, after cancer and heart disease.

Looking at the numbers, it initially seems like there's been a rise in medical errors, when in fact, there has only been improvement in reporting them. While a zero error percentage is not likely attainable, progress can be made in this area.

In order to reduce medical errors, we have to make it possible for them to be discussed in an atmosphere that is not punitive.

First, we have to acknowledge that these things happen, instead of sweeping them under the rug. Second, we have to provide a safe harbor and a safe zone for people to discuss it. At Ochsner, there's a system for reporting errors anonymously so that more facts can come to light. An important requirement is not to blame the individual for an unintentional, isolated mistake, but to improve the system of care that will allow all healthcare providers to succeed going forward.

It's incredibly rare for a doctor to harm a patient intentionally. Still, when mistakes happen, healthcare providers are often too afraid of being punished to admit the mistake. This was the situation in the airline industry many years ago. Pilots were punished if they accumulated too many near misses, and they underreported them so that they could continue flying. The underreporting prevented others from learning from the issues that led to the near miss and air traffic fatalities accumulated. To remedy this, the Aviation Safety Reporting System (ASRS) was created as a confidential information-gathering service run out of NASA. Once the pilots realized that there were in fact no punitive actions for reporting errors, the volume of reporting errors skyrocketed, and systems were put in place to improve aviation safety. Today, flying is the safest mode of transportation, with fewer than three accidents occurring for every one million departures.

Imagine the solutions we could find and the best practices that could be developed if the medical field fostered a similar environment that welcomed honest discussion. There ought to be a way to post, "This patient experienced a medical error. This is what the mistake cost."

That way, we can learn from the mistake and put in place checks and balances to prevent it from happening again. In other words, use the mistake to make the system stronger without relying on individual fallibility. A stronger health system will prevent millions of future mistakes.

The outgoing model of this industry can be characterized as multiple healthcare silos, where the financial incentive is based on the volume of patients seen. Each healthcare silo, made up of doctors and care teams, holds valuable information about the patient that is generally difficult to obtain if you practice outside the silo. Since patients often receive care among different specialists, they likely interact with multiple healthcare silos, and care from the patient's perspective is fragmented and uncoordinated. Mistakes made are often underreported and rarely transmitted to other participants within the silo, much less outside the silo. Outcomes including clinical events as well as quality of life and patient satisfaction are not measured, and one's best method of judging quality is word of mouth.

The incoming model of our industry focuses on quality, accountability, and care coordination with a high reliance on measured outcomes including patient satisfaction. Payment to doctors and hospitals will be based on outcomes, not services. Communication between provider organizations will become paramount, and fragmentation and poor coordination will be exposed and financially penalized. It will be difficult for small physician practices to survive, and over time they will be consumed into larger group practices or hospital networks. Shared information systems will improve communication, and patients will have more access to quality metrics, costs, and patient ratings of prospective doctors and hospitals. Diagnostics, procedures, and other forms of medical services will be commoditized and will be awarded to those who demonstrate the best quality and cost at the highest satisfaction and access.

As in other industries, the individual consumer will hold the information necessary to make the best decision. Those delivery systems that truly focus on quality, cost, and access from the lens of the consumer will prosper. The good news for all of us is that the healthcare consumer wins big. The future is bright.

CHAPTER 5

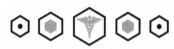

Patient Engagement and the Reduction of Healthcare Costs

P recision medicine is revolutionizing modern healthcare as well as our healthcare system. Precision medicine proposes healthcare that is customized and tailored to each individual in regard to medical decisions, prescriptions, treatments, and so on. It refers to the application of various gaming, education, and marketing theories to healthcare.

Companies like Netflix or Amazon provide each customer with unique recommendations based on previous purchases, current search results, and so forth. Similarly, precision medicine takes several factors into consideration before providing the patient with treatment options.

Applying these practices within the medical field ensures a patient's age, health, weight, gender, previous and current medications, lifestyle, socioeconomic status, and so on are all taken into account before creating and implementing a unique treatment plan. This is particularly powerful in changing the healthcare industry because it facilitates patient engagement and empowerment.

In the previous chapter, we talked about how the healthcare system can improve in regard to physician-patient relationships. An important component of such relationships involves empowering patients so that they aren't heavily and constantly relying on a doctor.

Now is the best time to advocate for this type of self-care because we are currently in the "Gutenberg moment" of the medical industry. In the same way that Gutenberg invented the printing press and made it possible for more people to read and access information for themselves, innovations in medical technology are now making it easier for people to access their own healthcare records and information.

Two or three thousand years ago, people had to go to the oracles in order to gain knowledge. In medieval times, only the monks could read and write, while the majority of people were illiterate.

In 1440, when the printing press came along, everything changed. By 1440, scholars estimate that there were approximately 30,000 books and manuscripts in circulation. Just sixty years later, in 1500, there were an estimated 12 million.

In terms of medical information, we're at the same kind of inflection point. The patient goes in for a visit, pays a fee, and then must assume that the doctor is providing accurate information, since the medical jargon that is often used is difficult for most to understand. Generally, patients don't even have access to their own medical records. The way that the system has been set up does not allow for transparency. *The doctor serves as the information gatekeeper, the only one who can collect, interpret, and distribute data.*

Now the roles are rapidly changing. Patients can collect medical information off the Internet and have access to biologic information about themselves without a doctor's intervention.

In Arizona and California, individuals can order their own lab work. Of course, it's now the patient's responsibility to interpret the data because a doctor is not being paid to do so. Still, patients can go online and talk to a professional about the test results. Patients can even send the reports to someone who knows how to interpret the information, while still others can learn how to understand lab reports and test results for themselves.

Individuals now have access to biologic information about themselves that they could not have gotten at any other time. The same is true about blood pressure, oxygen levels, and several other important health factors. For many of these data, individuals don't need to visit a lab for tests since they can receive the information they need from equipment purchased in a store or online. People are able to do tests for strep throat or urinary tract infections through over-the-counter products.

The result is that physicians are becoming commoditized—who needs a doctor for basic things when you can do so much yourself? It is becoming increasingly apparent that this is the direction that the medical field is headed, which is of concern to many doctors.

For example, while individuals have always had the legal right to request a copy of their medical records, most medical practices usually charge upwards of $50 and take about three weeks to prepare the documents for the patient. With the technology that is available now, this method is no longer appropriate.

As everything is electronic, complete medical records can be emailed within minutes and at no extra cost for the doctor. Though an objective approach views this as a more efficient method of sharing patient information, this type of process isn't being adopted across the board.

A similar concern seems to underlie the implementation of the patient portal. While a patient portal is approached as a quick and efficient way for patients to view their records, it implies a limited amount of access. The basic mindset of the portal is highly paternalistic in that the doctor has all of the access, but provides the patient with a limited amount of information that has been deemed appropriate for the patient to see. Why shouldn't patients have access to all of their information?

Individuals don't have a "portal" at a bank—they have access to every bit of financial information in regard to their accounts. Otherwise, they would pull their money out and go elsewhere. Still, the medical community thinks that patients should be grateful that they have a glimpse through a peephole into information that is rightfully theirs.

Let's look at this survey examining the level of access to electronic medical records viewed from the lens of the patient versus the physician.

Level of Access to One's Electronic Medical Record

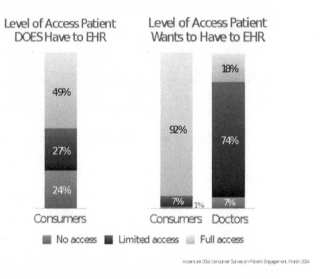

Level of Access Patient DOES Have to EHR

49%
27%
24%

Consumers

Level of Access Patient Wants to Have to EHR

18%
92%
74%
7%   1%   7%

Consumers   Doctors

■ No access   ■ Limited access   Full access

Accenture 2016 Consumer Survey on Patient Engagement, March 2016

Not only is there a divergence of opinion regarding access, but that divergence is getting worse, not better.

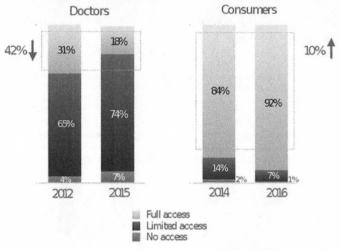

Growing Gap among Patients and Doctors on "Full Access" to EHRs

Doctors | Consumers

Doctors: 42%↓ — 31% / 65% / 4% (2012); 18% / 74% / 7% (2015)

Consumers: 10%↑ — 84% / 14% / 2% (2014); 92% / 7% / 1% (2016)

Full access
Limited access
No access

Accenture 2016 Consumer Survey on Patient Engagement. March 2016

The doctor's job should not be to control patient information, but to help patients understand the information in depth. While the concern at times is that bombarding patients with too much information up front can cause panic, the patient's reaction is largely affected by the manner in which the doctor communicates the information—as we saw in the story of my mother-in-law.

As the medical industry continues to progress, patients will have even more access to information about themselves, whether it be blood tests, strep tests, urinary infection tests, or even their genomes. Doctors need to begin changing their approach to match the information era—it's no longer the case that the doctor knows best.

As this open medical information model and patient empowerment spreads, patients will find that they are no longer limited by geography in terms of finding the best people to interpret their information. The expert needed to interpret certain genomic information may be based in San Diego while the patient lives hundreds of miles away; *distance is no longer an obstacle to receiving expert advice.*

Instead of worrying about a loss of income or control, many doctors are choosing to stay up to date on their specialties so that they are the experts that patients seek.

To adjust to this changing landscape, doctors should be able to diagnose and point patients to the appropriate individuals to initiate treatments. I might diagnose a person with a certain cancer, but I'm not an oncologist. I wouldn't be able to confidently prescribe a patient diagnosed with cancer with a solid treatment plan. It would be my job, however, to get the patient to the people who are the best suited for the specific oncology needs at hand. This will be the role of the doctor going forward.

We will need just as many, if not more, doctors than we have today. The role of the personal physician will never disappear, but it is going to continue to change radically.

The availability of medical information from live human beings via the Internet is another area in which we'll begin to notice rapid growth. Patients can have access to great medical care from a physician anywhere in the world in the middle of the night, from the comfort of their own home.

If your child wakes up at midnight with a sore throat and you do a rapid strep screen yourself that comes out positive, you can go to M.D. Live and meet with a doctor on your computer. After explaining the situation, the doctor can recommend the best therapy and send in a prescription along with what to do if your child isn't feeling better within forty-eight hours.

You're not making an appointment, you're not called in to sit in a waiting room, you don't have to wait two days to get in, and you no longer have to take time off from work. The process is more efficient and the child actually gets healthier faster because medicine becomes on-demand.

Of course there will be issues that aren't as simple as strep throat, but online information will still prove invaluable to patients. For example, if a woman notices a lump in her breast, the doctor will then order a mammogram. The patient will now be able to evaluate the cost of getting a mammogram done at various imaging centers. Certainly there will be sites that provide customer ratings to accompany the description of each center. The patient will have complete transparency and see that it's $150 at one center, but only $75 at another, which even has better ratings both from patients and doctors.

While doctors have a moral responsibility to provide each patient with the best possible care, the fee model that exists today means that businesspeople, not doctors, are making life-and-death decisions about medical care.

Any insurer, healthcare provider, or hospital can claim to be patient-centric, but many times they are profit-centric. The decision makers within the healthcare industry have not taken the Hippocratic oath and are not involved with patients on a one-on-one level as most doctors are. The businesspeople are making decisions from a purely financial standpoint.

My hope is that the "Gutenberg revolution" I'm describing in these pages will not leave this process unscathed either. Supreme Court Justice Louis Brandeis wrote a century ago, "Sunlight is the best disinfectant." Empowering patients with information and access to experts across the globe is a great example of such sunlight.

While businesspeople and some doctors may react to the changing landscape with fear, this Gutenberg moment also serves as a market opportunity for healthcare product companies. It's all about shifting your focus and adjusting your role, and not about trying to hold onto something that is slipping away.

Today, you can find more than 200,000 health and wellness or fitness-related apps available for sale. A study found that about half were not useful, and that many don't provide good advice or offer anything of value. Still, there are plenty that are quite excellent.

A lot of the money that currently flows to doctors will be increasingly diverted to companies that make better apps. If you have diabetes, you may only see your doctor every three months. Or you can look at your statistics using any number of excellent diabetes apps. If you see green, you know you're under good diabetes control. If you see yellow, you know you could be doing better and need to up your game. This is extremely helpful, and it's information that a doctor simply cannot provide you in real time.

PATIENT ACTIVATION

An interesting phenomenon along these lines is called "patient activation." Very simply, the patients who come into the doctor's office with a stack of articles they've printed off the Internet are often viewed as an annoyance by the doctor, but now it's been statistically proven that those individuals are much more actively involved with their healthcare. Those patients are much more likely to comply with whatever a doctor says, and as a result, those patients are more actively engaged with their healthcare teams.

By contrast, a patient who is not very engaged often does not adhere to a medication or lifestyle regimen. As a result, *these individuals are more likely to encounter mistakes in their diagnosis and treatment.*

Interestingly, insurance companies are actually excited about the concept of patient activation, probably because it lays less of a financial responsibility on the insurer. They would love to have a million insured people on the books who are highly activated—it's insuring people who aren't likely to need expensive services because activation makes you healthier.

A system that empowers patients to take better care of themselves improves healthcare outcomes. At this time, the majority of health systems are still learning to go from volume to value. They're asking, "How do I become a high-quality healthcare system?"

On its face, the question is absurd because they should already be meeting that standard, if not surpassing it. That's why the healthcare system is in need of change—doctors have been paid for volume, so they've never had to worry about creating value. They've never had to worry about activation.

Patients keep coming back to the hospital because there is no other option available, and the healthcare system keeps making more money. That's how it's always been. Now, doctors have to worry about how the patient feels and how the patient is going to rate the doctor—patient satisfaction and patient activation.

What kinds of outcomes are we getting right now? There was a study published a dozen years ago in the *New England Journal of Medicine* that looked at medical management in terms of whether patients were on the right medicines for diabetes, COPD, high blood pressure, and similar chronic conditions.

It turns out that only 25–60 percent of the patients were on the right therapy—as many as 50–60 percent were not. *You had almost a 50 percent chance that you weren't on the right therapy if you had a chronic condition in the United States.*

As a result, healthcare providers and insurers are much more concerned about process measures than ever before. Process measures usually lead to good results. The trouble is not just that we've been misdiagnosing and providing the wrong prescriptions. We're also measuring the wrong things. Process measures, which have been the focus in the medical community for years, are terrific, but what really matter are the outcomes the process measures are trying to influence.

In the medical industry, outcomes occur in three tiers. The first is very simple—did you live or die? Was the operation a success or a failure?

The second tier is, what's the disutility here? You lived, but now you have to come back to the hospital fifteen times to treat the infection the doctor gave you or the mistake he made when he left a sponge in your stomach. That's disutility.

The third tier is that you had a knee operation because you had pain in your knee, but a year has gone by and you still can't walk any further than you did before surgery. So the knee operation was technically a success but worthless to the patient because the quality of life did not improve. These are the real outcomes. Process measures and standards do help, but they're only a small step on the way to what we need to measure and accomplish.

People have to be able to say, "I'm going to go see Dr. Milani for my knee replacement because he's got the lowest disutility rate. He's got the highest survival rate. And when you look at outcomes for improving the quality of life, reducing pain, and improving walking distance for patients with knee replacements, he's got the best statistics." That's where the world is headed—patients will be empowered to have that information instead of simply being resigned to who is local and available.

The gold standard is to have all healthcare providers using a universal set of agreed-upon outcome measures. This includes the patients contributing to the conversation with their experience and opinions, the same way they do on Expedia when they rate a hotel. People spend a lot of time adding comments to those sites with specific details. Or they'll simply write, "I had a great experience." It's easy to understand why doctors and hospitals fear being judged on outcomes and not just on process, and this is precisely what I mean by the difference between measuring volume and measuring value.

One of the most important pieces of the puzzle for delivering better outcomes is the mobile phone. By 2020, over 80 percent of the world population, even sub-Saharan Africa, will have a smartphone. This means that practically everyone on the planet can be reached by technology that pings them a week or a month after a hospitalization or doctor visit to ask, "Hey, Sam, how are things going today? How far are you walking today?" These things will be automated and built into healthcare.

Phones also provide remarkable amounts of data, as long as privacy is maintained. There was a study at MIT where they asked students living in the dorm during flu season a few simple questions. They had to answer the questions every day, via the smartphones MIT provided for them. "Do you have fever? Do you feel sick today? Are you stressed? Do you have a runny nose or sore throat?"

The deal was this—if they answered the questions every day, which would only take them a few seconds, they would get $1 for each time they answered. At the end of this study, they got to keep the smartphone.

The application in the phone not only gathered this information, but it also indicated the distance each student walked or traveled on a given day, how many phone calls they made, how many different people they contacted, and when they made the phone calls.

While the application could not overhear the calls or determine with whom they spoke, it would spit out the data that John Doe called seventeen different people today and spoke for an average length of two minutes. As a result, the app was able to accurately predict when they were stressed and exactly when they were sick solely based on their activity and telephone use. They were actually able to predict illness based off of ubiquitous data obtained from any smartphone. So applications not only give patients information—they can help providers as well.

These innovations don't work perfectly yet. Google Flu Trends is an example of a big data project whose time has not yet come. Google Flu Trends completely missed the major 2013 flu epidemic, so the information from this service is no longer available to the people.

On a personal level, these innovations mean that anything you're doing requires careful, thoughtful analysis. Amazon knows when you're interested in taking a vacation because it studies your patterns. Based on those patterns Amazon understands that they don't have to be right 100 percent of the time, but they will be right more than they're wrong, and the vacation-related offerings they make will be of some interest to the customer.

In medicine, it's the same thing. We don't have to be right 100 percent of the time. We can get people more and more information and they can give you certain guidelines. The outcome is progress in the system and improvement for individual lives.

Patient satisfaction now matters to doctors in a way that it hasn't in the past. We want patients to be fully engaged, we want their outcomes to be excellent, and we can get great ratings because of it. If the patient and the doctor are working together, everybody wins—the insurer, the doctor, and the patient. Disease control actually improves and chronic diseases diminish in severity.

In our current healthcare system, 86 percent of all dollars go to chronic problems such as cancer, heart disease, stroke, diabetes, high blood pressure, and high cholesterol.[89] Patient activation has the potential to decrease 86 percent of expenditures—think about the number of people who will experience an improved quality of life because of improvements made through their own empowerment.

89 "Chronic Disease Prevention and Health Promotion." Centers for Disease Control and Prevention. November 14, 2016. https://www.cdc.gov/chronicdisease/.

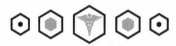

CHAPTER 6

Empowering Patients to Take Care of Themselves

The previous chapter largely focused on patient activation because patient activation leads to patient engagement.

Patient engagement is arguably one of the most important factors in improving health and wellness, though methods for achieving it are left out of the curriculum at most medical schools.

The term patient engagement is used to describe the concept of patients taking the lead in their own healthcare. The reality in today's world is that the patient—not the doctor, hospital, or medical professional online—must be his or her own primary healthcare provider. That puts a lot of responsibility on the part of the patient, and rightly so; after all, there is no benefit to visiting a doctor and receiving a diagnosis or prescription if the patient then does not implement the treatment or plan of action.

A patient's health certainly won't improve, and will probably continue to decline, if there is a lack of follow-through. A doctor cannot do anything beyond offering expert advice, providing prescriptions, and recommending a plan of action. With this in mind, the medical community is then tasked with answering this question: How can we get patients to realize that our function is not to rescue people, but instead to put them on a path where they can take care of themselves?

Sparking patient engagement is an in-depth process, and we must start with small, measurable, and realistic goals, not a list of dozens of changes to implement. If you want to measure patient engagement on a one-to-five scale, and the patient is at a one, the lowest level, then we must first try to move the patient to a two. If they're at a two, let's get them to a three. What we don't want to do is try to rush a patient from a one to a four. It's not realistic or sustainable, and if patients feel that the plan is impossible, they are far less likely to try.

I like the analogy of travel: If you live in California and are headed to Hawaii, you first need to know how to get to the airport before you fly to the island. Though getting to Hawaii from California is a much longer and more complex process, breaking it down into small, measurable goals increases the likelihood of establishing lasting success.

The necessity of implementing such as process is particularly apparent in chronic issues like diabetes or high blood pressure. It's the doctor's job to teach the necessary skills in a way that makes sense to the patient. It is then the patient's job to pay attention, ask questions, and apply these skills moving forward.

One of the major research studies on the topic of patient engagement shows that patients with the lowest activation or engagement scores incur healthcare costs up to 21 percent higher than those with the highest levels.[90] But it's not just financial costs. The reality is that people who don't take care of themselves are going to have even more health problems down the line.

Let's say you come to the hospital for whatever reason, and you get a plan of action when you're discharged. If you don't follow it, you'll likely be back in the hospital within thirty days. Once you're back in the hospital, you're more likely to have other problems since you're also exposing yourself to iatrogenic issues as well as poor coordination between healthcare providers. You're going to a cardiologist, you see your primary care doctor, and then you're in the hospital. Who's coordinating your medications? Who's coordinating your treatment plan? You could suffer a health consequence due to poor provider communication. This happens all the time, and it especially happens to those patients with a low level of engagement.

---

90   Hibbard, Judith H., and Jessica Greene. "Patients With Lower Activation Associated With Higher Costs; Delivery Systems Should Know Their Patients' Scores." Health Affairs. February 01, 2013. http://content.healthaffairs.org/content/32/2/216.full.

Before we can implement change, we must understand why patients aren't engaged. For some, it is a lack of long-term focus in life because of more immediate problems in their lives. Socioeconomics, mental health, and various other factors play an important role in patient engagement. For example, someone who is preoccupied with finding a way to pay for groceries is unlikely to be immediately concerned with having a yearly physical. A patient suffering from depression who has become isolated from others isn't necessarily suicidal, but is disengaged to the point of neglecting self-care and health management.

There's a higher prevalence of disengagement among less educated and less affluent populations. In lower socioeconomic classes, you may not have immediate access to experts, and for many, it's nearly impossible to even get the time off of work to go in for a doctor visit.

Aside from cases that involve factors such as socioeconomic status and mental health, patient engagement generally begins with the doctor. Doctors are trained to make diagnoses and then share the proper therapeutic plan with the patient. Beyond that, doctors generally believe that they have fulfilled their part, and if the patient doesn't follow through on the proposed plan, it's the patient's fault. Now that physicians are becoming increasingly responsible for patient outcomes, there is a genuine interest in learning how healthcare providers can have an impact on patient engagement. The problem is that doctors have not been trained in methods of fostering patient engagement or in recognizing obstacles to patient engagement.

There are, however, plenty of simple steps a doctor can take in order to facilitate patient engagement. If the goal is to move a patient diagnosed with high blood pressure from scale one to scale two, asking the patient to take their blood pressure at home would be a step in the right direction. The doctor could suggest the patient purchase a blood pressure cuff and request that the patient simply take his blood pressure once a week, which would then be sent to the doctor. If the doctor explains this thoroughly and asks the patient to participate in this, it is very likely that the patient will follow through. The moral of the story: patient engagement begins with small steps.

Doctors play a large role in patient engagement, and understanding this will help find solutions to patient disengagement. For example, one of the biggest predictors of readmission to the hospital for patients with heart failure is simply whether the patient is willing to weigh himself daily. It's not about trying to get the patient to lose weight, but just to check if the patient has gained two or three pounds overnight. One of the surest indicators of heart failure is when patients gain fluid overnight, which is why doctors ask the patient to step onto the scale in the morning. Many patients resist because they don't want to admit to or be reprimanded for eating or drinking poorly the day before. Patients may not realize that the daily weigh-ins are about seeing if you are at risk for exacerbating heart failure so that we can do something about it *today*. If the doctor doesn't explain this, the patient will likely be resistant to participating.

Open and honest communication initiated by the doctor is extremely powerful in fostering patient engagement.

People want to be involved in their own healthcare, but they need to be empowered through education and communication. According to several national surveys, patients are absolutely thirsty for a high level of engagement in their own healthcare. We see statistics indicating that more than nine out of ten individuals want to be involved in their healthcare decision-making. This is why health and wellness applications are one of the fastest-growing segments in the app industry. While this isn't a fair assessment, because socioeconomic status again plays a role in having access to smartphones and health and wellness apps, the numbers still show that a significant portion of the population want to be intimately involved in their own healthcare; technology is an obvious gateway for that involvement.

As we see that sometimes it's not a matter of patient engagement, the challenge can also be as simple as getting patients to alter their expectations. For example, people come to the doctor with a common cold or virus and expect an antibiotic for treatment, not realizing that classic colds and ear infections don't respond to antibiotics since they aren't bacterial in nature.

Unfortunately, many patients get upset if they don't get a prescription for antibiotics because they believe that antibiotics are necessary in order to get well. Again, this is a matter of communicating honestly with patients, and providing them evidence (such as a brochure) that antibiotics not only won't help, but could cause harm. The Centers for Disease Control (CDC) have created educational materials for patients on the importance of avoiding inappropriate antibiotics, and we are using them at Ochsner in our antibiotic stewardship campaign. These resources are available on the web to anyone: http://

www.cdc.gov/getsmart/community/materials-references/print-materials/adults/index.html

Empowering patients to engage in their own healthcare is extremely complex and difficult because it's a matter of changing people's behaviors. We are finding that the fear of being ranked poorly relative to their peers is a greater motivator in changing doctors' behaviors than the promise of a monetary reward. Doctors dread being ranked poorly. When you've got a system in place that lists how everybody is doing relative to other doctors, it motivates most doctors to try harder.

Interestingly, monetary rewards generally do seem to motivate patients to engage in behavioral changes. The administrator of a large healthcare plan once mentioned that when the deductible for a group went up from $500 a year to $2,000 per year, many of the patients stopped going to the doctor for routine issues for which they would have to pay out of pocket. Still, getting patients to change their behavior is sometimes as simple as helping them to see the connection between cause and effect.

Let's return to the example of a patient with heart failure, a condition where the heart cannot meet the metabolic demands of the body. The doctor will say to the patient with low activation, "Take it easy on those potato chips, those pickles, and the Chinese food. There's too much salt in them." But maybe the patient doesn't fully comprehend and as a result must go back to the hospital relatively soon.

The doctor then tells the patient, "You have to weigh yourself every day on a scale that feeds me the results. If I notice that your weight has gone up two or three pounds, I'm going to call you. I may ask, 'What did you eat yesterday?' If I call you three or four times, eventually you'll finally get the point—you ate Chinese food, which has a lot of salt, which meant that you retained fluid, which meant that your weight went up, which signaled that you are at risk for exacerbating your heart failure." The doctor hopes that eventually the patient will understand the correlation and that those results will motivate behavioral change—and statistically, it does. Sometimes we see that it's just about helping people connect the dots.

Many doctors don't actively engage in practices to increase patient engagement because they may be unaware when a patient has a low level of engagement. Our medical school system is still steeped in the traditional model of teaching about disease and treatment, and doctors are typically given little education about behavior modification. It may be that the faculty simply doesn't know the issue or is unable to change the curriculum, which means that it will be another generation before medical school changes in a meaningful way. Doctors are going to have to receive training about patient engagement as well as behavior modification. Until behavioral modification techniques are taught in medical school, a powerful first step would be setting up such training sessions in hospitals.

It's usually even harder for patients to get a clear sense of what they're supposed to do, even if they want to be engaged, when they are admitted to a hospital. Nurses and doctors come and go and the patient often is confused who his or her doctor is. A recent study revealed that only 32 percent of hospitalized patients could correctly name even one of their hospital physicians.[91] The doctor might come while making rounds when your spouse or family member isn't there, and the patient might remember some of what the doctor said but is not likely to remember all of it.

How does a patient assimilate such important information when feeling emotional and scared? In a perfect world, we give the patient a tablet. Not a pill—a tablet like an iPad, and the patient can easily find a photo and short biography of the doctor as well as the nurse. The tablet will also display a listing of the medications the patient is taking along with links to learn more about the disease for which the patient is admitted, test results, and a schedule for their stay.

We actually have a program in place called the "Optimal Hospital." In the Optimal Hospital unit, we have fifteen beds, which means that if the average person stays two or three days in the hospital, you'll turn the beds over two or three times a week. That means thirty to forty patients may come through in an average week.

In that first week, those patients turned on their tablets and looked up their medications 363 times. They looked at their schedules 161 times. They got information about who's on their care team 94 times, viewed results of their tests 86 times, and looked at prescribed education files 51 times.

---

91   O'Leary, Kevin J., Nita Kulkarni, Matthew P. Landler, Jiyeon Jeon, Katherine J. Hahn, Katherine M. Englert, and Mark V. Williams. "Hospitalized Patients' Understanding of Their Plan of Care." Mayo Clinic Proceedings. January 2010. https://www.ncbi.nlm.nih.gov/pmc/articles/PMC2800283/.

It makes sense that the average American visits a doctor three times a year, but spends more than fifty-two hours on the Internet looking at health information.[92] The beauty of this system is that when you've got all that information on your iPad there, you can actually record the conversation when the doctor comes in for rounds and play it back to yourself, your spouse, or your caregiver as often as you like. Doctors are actually in favor of this sort of technology because they would rather you have all your people present so everyone's questions are answered and they don't have to come back and repeat the same speech over and over again.

The single best behavior change program is cardiac rehabilitation. I've written dozens of papers on this topic. The simple reality is that patients actually make each other better. You might have one patient who's a construction worker and another who is a famous writer. They have nothing in common—they have never met, and they never would have socialized because they live completely different lives. Yet the construction worker has been in the program for six weeks and it's the famous writer's first day, so the construction worker is going to help the writer. She's going to say, "Look, the pain will last a little longer, but it'll get better if you do this and do that."

It's remarkable how people from different experiences will bond over the treatment of their common illness. The socialization makes all the difference. The program would likely

92   Loechner, Jack. "Three Doctor Visits and 52 Hours of Online Health Search A Year." September 25, 2013. https://www.mediapost.com/ publications/article/209665/three-doctor-visits-and-52-hours-of-online-health.html.

succeed if we had robots treating people, even though we have truly great nurses, because it's the social interactions among the patients that is key. Teaching each other about the different levels of the disease process and what they've learned along the way makes all the difference. It's even more meaningful because the doctor may never have had the diabetes, cancer, or heart attack that the patient has suffered, but the other patients recognize what they're going through. It's that sense of empathy and teamwork towards a common goal that has such a profound impact.

We are continually finding such examples of improved processes and solutions to obstacles that loom over improved healthcare. Yet, advancements seem to be coming slowly. Why don't things change more quickly? One reason is that in any endeavor, when one tries new things, one will experience a high failure rate. Not everything new works, and, as we've discussed in previous chapters, the culture in the medical community, as in most industries, is to punish failure.

We need to embrace what Thomas Edison said: "I have not failed. I've just found 10,000 ways that won't work."

Many of the greatest innovations in business have taken place by the creation of skunkworks—secret facilities that companies create, practically off the books, so that their best people can innovate fulltime without fear of being punished for failure. Lockheed created the first jet in the United States through a skunkworks solution. GM created the Corvette the same way, behind locked doors that the bean counters could not penetrate.

The medical field is, of course, different from these examples because we are dealing with people's lives and their wellbeing. Still, before we can get patients to change their mentality about engagement, we in the medical community have to change our mentality about embracing failure. How can we ask our patients to be innovative in terms of their attitude toward their healthcare if we in the medical community, from hospitals to medical schools to frontline doctors' offices, refuse to innovate ourselves? Though it may be difficult for many doctors, we have to model the behavior that we want to encourage in our patients and show what a difference engagement really does make.

CHAPTER 7

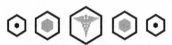

The Five Fastest Ways to Control Healthcare Costs and Save Lives

Revolutionizing our current healthcare system by triggering patient activation and implementing more patient-centric processes echoes the overall theme of this book. Exploring how we can empower patients and physicians through revised approaches and the use of health-and-wellness-centered IT will enable both to form strong partnerships that pave the way to improved healthcare.

This chapter builds on this theme by exploring what I've identified as the five fastest ways to control healthcare costs and save lives: transparency, communication, volume to value, behavior change, and patient engagement.

Taking full advantage of new health-and-wellness-centered technologies will allow us to build on these five points and, ultimately, improve our healthcare system.

The Accenture survey presented in Chapter 5 states that roughly 50 percent of people in the United States have access to their electronic health records. The other half is divided in almost equal parts between people who have no access, and people who have partial access.

While legally, patients have always had full access to their own medical records, it generally takes extra money and a long wait time to receive the information requested. I believe that the reasoning behind the desire most physicians have of giving patients only partial access to their records is twofold. First, many physicians tend to want to filter information that their patients receive in order to curb the amount of questions they have to answer or details they have to give. As discussed previously, doctors are already rushed through patient visits and proper documentation processes, so the idea of spending an hour on the phone with each person who is confused by their records can be somewhat intimidating.

The second reason behind the push for limited access is also fear-based. Some doctors, especially the more inexperienced ones, may be concerned about someone finding a potential error in their work or documentation, so they would rather have as few eyes as possible on what they do. Until the healthcare industry changes its punitive response to mistakes and errors, most doctors are not going to want their patients to find issues or discrepancies in their medical records. By using issues as a means to finding solutions, instead of shaming doctors, we'll create stronger patient-physician relationships and increase the level of transparency in healthcare.

1. TRANSPARENCY

As we know, errors do occur all the time, so transparency is actually one of the five factors that I have identified as being able to lower costs and improve medical care.

A great example of how transparency can improve the healthcare industry can be seen through the OpenNotes Initiative. OpenNotes was a study that focused on 105 doctors sharing all their clinical notes with over nineteen thousand patients. It was initially met with some resistance, but researchers convinced enough doctors to participate, and it turned out to be wildly beneficial in multiple ways.

OpenNotes is able to save lives and reduce costs because it increases patient engagement, which we already know directly improves treatment outcomes. It also enables the patient to identify mistakes that may otherwise go undetected. The chart may read "diabetic," which the patient will know is a mistake since they've never been diagnosed with or displayed evidence of diabetes.

Patients frequently identify errors in their medical records by reading through the charts in OpenNotes. This helps avoid issues down the line when immediate care is needed. On a similar note, it helps with medical reconciliation in terms of ensuring prescription and treatment information is up to date.

Another great aspect of a system like OpenNotes is that it doesn't cost the patient or insurance company anything. The only thing that is needed to read the notes in OpenNotes is access to Electronic Medical Records (EMR) and a patient portal, which is something that most places are required to have anyway. There is so much interest in this idea of transparency that the OpenNotes Initiative has become more of a movement now, with about six million patients in the United States currently participating.

What's really exciting about OpenNotes is that patients and healthcare facilities seem equally invested in this approach. Harvard's Beth Israel, Geisinger Health System, Ochsner Health System, and the Department of Veterans Affairs are only some of the large players.

OpenNotes is an example of a very simple way that we're able to implement change within the healthcare system. Such changes ensure that patients are truly able to partner with their doctors in treating and preventing health issues. Transparency will control costs by engaging the patient, and it will save lives by catching errors before they become problems.

2. COMMUNICATION

Another one of the five fastest ways to lower costs and save lives is through communication. Research from the Joint Commission shows that 62 percent of accidental deaths and 80 percent of serious medical errors occur due to communication failures. These encompass communication between physicians, between a physician and a nurse, a physician and the patient, and even delayed communication or a lack of communication overall. It is estimated that the current economic impact of communication inefficiencies in the United States alone is $11.2 billion annually.

There are also issues related to medical records that aren't transferred and communications between two different hospitals or medical centers. This may partly be due to the fact that sending information back and forth has never been an easy or simple process. Another issue is that some patients have hundreds of pages of medical documentation and now the hospital or medical clinic has to go through it all to find the ten pieces of information they really need in the moment. So communication failures don't necessarily mean lack of communication, but rather a processing inefficiency.

What we are seeing in the research and by taking a look at the process is that improving communication methods can drastically improve treatment outcomes, save lives, and reduce costs spent on unnecessary medication, treatment, and error. There are improvements being made, such as continuity of care documents (CCDs) that are being used to transfer medical information between clinics and hospitals, but there is still room for improvement in this department.

3. VOLUME TO VALUE

The third from my list of the five fastest ways to reduce costs and improve outcomes ties back to an earlier chapter: volume to value. The medical industry today is moving from a volume business to a value-based business, and that, in and of itself, will control costs and save lives.

Instead of focusing on the amount of treatment provided or the number of prescriptions written, we are beginning to value the actual outcomes. Michael Porter of Harvard Business School wrote about moving toward a value-based system in the *New England Journal of Medicine*. His essay covers how to define and determine value, and then breaks the concept of measuring value into the three tiers we discussed in Chapter 5.

1. Whether the patient lives, or the degree of health or recovery.
2. The process of recovery. This includes the time to recovery and time to normal work activities. This also includes what is referred to as the disutility of care or treatment, which refers to any complications or adverse events occurring after implementing the procedure, medication, or treatments.
3. The sustainability of health and includes whether quality of life is actually improved.

While there are several variables at play here, Porter's essay exhibits the increasing level of awareness that the volume to value model is receiving.

The volume to value measurements basically come down to life, death, disutility, and quality of life. If we're using these measurements then we can truly measure outcomes, all of which plays an important role in lowering overall costs and saving lives.

As discussed earlier, when doctors are held accountable for the value that they bring, which becomes public knowledge amongst their peers, they are much more likely to implement change. While doctors may see fewer patients each day, the extra time they spend with each patient will increase the value of their work, thereby improving the care that patients receive. This is turn lowers costs and potentially saves lives, which positively impacts revenue to the health delivery system.

4. BEHAVIORAL CHANGE

Previous examples have truly shown how behavioral change leads to reduced costs and improved healthcare outcomes. Let's look at another example: Peripheral Arterial Disease (PAD) refers to the condition of blockages that occur in leg arteries. Blockages in the heart arteries may be asymptomatic if the patient is walking from one room to the next, but if the patient is going for a longer walk at a slightly brisker pace, he may start having angina, which is due to not getting enough blood flow to the heart muscle. The patient's body is requiring more oxygen and energy, and the more he exercises, the more he needs. The symptoms generally manifest as chest discomfort and difficulty breathing. The same is true of blockages in the arteries of the legs. If I have blockages there, then I can probably walk from here to the bathroom, but maybe not. If I go beyond a certain point, I'm going to experience enough pain in my legs to make me stop. This limits the patient's quality of life.

So what can the doctor do? Well, you want to improve their walking distance, which is a quality of life issue. Currently, the only drug that can help with this is called cilostazol, and the average wholesale price for that drug in the United States is about $2,600 a year. This is very expensive, but the patient will see that walking distance on average will improve by 50 percent. Cilostazol doesn't work in all cases, and depending on where the blockages are, some patients will need bypass surgery or stenting. Bypass surgery and stenting are two procedures that may improve the blood flow to the patient's legs, but both are pretty expensive, though most insurance companies will cover the cost.

It is surprising, then, that insurance companies generally won't cover the cost of supervised exercise, which, according to some research, is proven to improve patient mobility by 150 percent on average. To pay out of pocket, and this may be an overestimate, supervised exercise might cost $1,800. The question that usually arises here is why not exercise alone? Why does it need to be supervised?

When patients begin to exercise in light of an illness, injury, or disease, most tend to stop as soon as they feel pain or discomfort. During supervised exercise sessions, the patient is being reassured that the pain is normal while receiving motivational coaching and positive reinforcement that pushes patients to continue exercising. The little bit of extra exertion during exercise is what causes new blood vessels to grow, so patients are actually creating their own bypass and manufacturing new blood vessels naturally.

There was another study done on patients who were on the edge of being diabetic.[93] It's a progressive effect: the patient

93   Diabetes Prevention Program Research Group. "Reduction in the Incidence of Type 2 Diabetes with Lifestyle Intervention or Metmorfin." New England Journal of Medicine. February 7, 2002. https://www.nejm.org/doi/full/10.1056/NEJMoa012512#t=article.

usually goes from normal to slightly abnormal, then from slightly abnormal to being on the edge of diabetes, and finally being fully diabetic.

The study focused on people diagnosed as prediabetic and the group was randomly separated into three groups. One group was given a placebo, another group received the diabetic medication metformin, and the third group received a very strongly focused behavioral change intervention.

Being equal thirds, the worst in terms of health improvements was seen in the group that received the placebo. The group that was given metformin maintained better health than the first group, but was outperformed by the group that had received the behavioral change intervention.

Behavior beats a lot of other things in a lot of conditions, but it takes time and effort. Behavioral change is the greatest way to save lives. It wins in every aspect, it saves on costs, it saves lives, and it improves quality of life.

So if it's proven that if you exercise a little bit more and eat a little bit healthier, why don't people do that?

Let's ask the reverse question.

When a Pepsi commercial comes on the TV, why do you want to go drink a Pepsi? When you see a McDonald's commercial come on with the fries and drink, why not go buy McDonald's?

There are a lot of counterforces. The writing on the cigarette package says, "This will kill you." Yet we see people buying cigarettes and smoking all the time. The question is, why do people take actions that harm themselves when they know full well they don't have to?

The answer is simple: because we're human.

No one is immune to advertising. We're either succumbing to the forces that Madison Avenue is delivering to us, or to that of the people that we surround ourselves with. Goldman Sachs ran several studies and found that the economic impact of behavioral modification and healthcare is "indefinitely large." Research indicates that 40 percent of one's health is determined by behavior. It's the single greatest contributing factor.

Adopting a healthier lifestyle will lower healthcare costs. Specifically, you're going to have less diabetes, strokes, heart attacks, blood pressure issues, and cholesterol problems. These are the chronic, behavior-related diseases that are bankrupting Americans. With behavior modification, you're either not getting the chronic disease that you would have gotten, or you're having more control over it, or you're on less medication than you would have been on before, and you're having fewer hospitalizations. Cost savings and health benefits are seen across the board.

5. Patient Engagement

Lastly, patient engagement is one of the five fastest ways to lower healthcare costs and save lives. The more the patient is engaged, the better the outcome is going to be.

With a high level of engagement, patients are more likely to take their medication appropriately and less likely to suffer complications, be readmitted to the hospital, and have errors take place in the healthcare system. All of this is because patients are taking a self-interest in the healthcare they are receiving. Moreover, patients who are engaged in their treatment are likely to be more discriminating about the physicians they work with, and less likely to work with doctors who won't share their clinical notes and so forth.

The real value is that you're going to be questioning things and you're going to be more active in your own healthcare process. This will lead to fewer errors and mistakes that could possibly occur.

Patient engagement includes getting into coordination of care. It's not only coordinated care among the healthcare team; it's coordinated care among the healthcare team with the most important person in the equation, the patient.

Traditionally, the most underutilized person in the equation is the patient, who happens to fill the most significant role in getting better, as we touched on in the previous chapter. The primary care physician really does need to be the co-captain of the ship along with the patient in order to ensure that the ship can chart through the complicated healthcare system.

The primary care physician also needs to guide the patient to the right specialist when appropriate, the right medication, and the right type of support system. Continuity of care also refers to staying with the same delivery system over time so that there is a continuous relationship. This allows healthcare providers to see what happened before and to not repeat mistakes while building on their prior knowledge of your condition, which will improve the treatment plan.

If a patient continuously goes to a different primary care physician, the relationship and the treatment plan are not going to be as intimate. Coordination of care is extremely important to maintaining patient engagement.

THE SOLUTION

Let's define the problem so that we can propose solutions. First, primary care doctors have very little time, yet much is expected from them. This is due to no fault of their own.

Second, they, like all physicians, have very little training in long-lasting behavior change. Today, they are not equipped with the tools needed to create long-lasting positive behavior change, which will surely help their patients, and they also have very little time to obtain these skills.

Third, the volume of current medical literature is exponential, making it impossible, even for specialists, to stay up to date with the research, literature, and best practices within their own trade.

In fact, there's actually been a study on the amount of work with which primary care physicians are tasked. The research shows that if primary care doctors were able to do everything they needed to do, it would take ten and a half hours a day just in the treatment of ten chronic diseases.[94]

It has already been made clear that doctors cannot do all that work aside from meeting with the patient. On top of that, doctors haven't been trained, they don't have the time or the resources to be able to pull this off, and that's why our healthcare system failing.

---

94   Ostbye, Truls, Kimberly S. H. Yarnall, Katrina M. Krause, Kathryn I. Pollak, Margaret Gradison, and J. Lloyd Michener. "Is There Time for Management of Patients With Chronic Diseases in Primary Care?" Annals of Family Medicine. May 2005. https://www.ncbi.nlm.nih.gov/pmc/articles/PMC1466884/.

Let's take a look at any other complicated big business, like a shoe manufacturer. If you're running the business, are you're going to look at your critical data (like supplies, expenses, and sales) four times a year to make sure that your business is heading in the right direction? More likely, you're focused on the details every day, how many pairs of what were sold, production costs, third-party vendors, advertisements, and so on. So you review that material every day, while reaching for specific markers quarterly. Why isn't a similar model applied to healthcare?

The current delivery model in our healthcare industry is built around acute problems. You break your arm, go to the hospital, sit in the waiting room, see a doctor, have your arm set, and then are asked to return in a week. When you return, you're told, "Things are looking good. I'll see you back in six weeks to take the cast off. Thank you."

This is absolutely a perfect system for colds, pneumonia, and broken bones. However, it's not designed for problems that change daily and are based on lifestyle, behavior, medication, and many other variables. As mentioned previously, 86 percent of our healthcare dollars are spent on such chronic issues. What is worse is that 75 percent of the deaths we see are related to these chronic issues as well. By adjusting the process so that behavior change is targeted, and the healthcare system monitors the disease condition on a real-time basis, we'll see huge benefits in health outcomes and huge cuts in healthcare costs.

Finding realistic ways of measuring the benefits of programs like supervised exercise and other activities or approaches that spark patient engagement and behavior change will document how these practices generate economic and social value for all involved. This value will serve as incentive for insurance companies, physicians, and medical schools to get on board. We are now seeing how programs that target behavior and lifestyle change also add value by saving lives and reducing costs. I believe it is inevitable that the healthcare industry will follow—to the benefit of patients and medical specialists alike.

CHAPTER 8

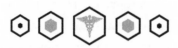

Big Data:
What's in it for you?

D ata science is a booming field in nearly every industry. Data scientists are experts in computational models, statistics, physics, and mathematics. While the more conventional and theoretical research within the healthcare industry is still conducted by physicians, scientists, and PhDs, data scientists are the professionals collecting and interpreting large volumes of data, which doesn't actually require expertise in healthcare.

Experts within healthcare identify a particular problem, or field of interest, and shape the research, while data scientists collect and interpret data for significant pieces of information.

By going outside of traditional clinical research, data scientists are helping to move the healthcare industry forward in a powerful way.

The healthcare industry needs data scientists, as many previous methods of obtaining information are no longer available to us. Traditionally, physicians physically wrote prescriptions and gave them to patients, and patients then had to go to a pharmacy to have the prescription filled. The number of prescriptions actually filled compared to the number written was known as the "fill rate," which was extremely valuable in identifying to the physician and payers which patients were not filling the prescriptions. This allowed the physician to then adequately plan a follow-up or intervention for the patient.

Today, this valuable information is not really available because electronic prescribing essentially creates a 100 percent fill rate. Before a patient walks out the front door of her physician's office, the prescription is already at the pharmacy and in the process of being filled.

What we need now are pickup rates, which seems simple enough, but that information is not actually available to us. When a prescription is picked up, that transaction is recorded, but not given to physicians or payers. This is an example of unutilized data: valuable information that we aren't making use of, even though it has the potential to save lives.

Big Data Use

Data generated in everyday medical practice goes largely unexplored, as is the case with the majority of data generated from most daily activities. Jeff Immelt, the CEO of GE, spoke about data that is generated in his industry, stating that a majority is not utilized. This is true in the healthcare industry as well; while data is interpreted for a specific purpose, a large portion of it, which can still provide valuable insights, is not being mined for additional value.

As I've mentioned in previous chapters, a recurring issue in healthcare is that many patients aren't regularly adhering to their medicines. Another significant issue is that patient adherence rates drop off dramatically. Only about one third of patients with even severe or life-threating problems, like recovering from a stroke or heart attack, continue taking their medications as prescribed after the first year. It's important to note that this is not always due to the side effects of the medications or the financial cost, but mainly we are seeing that patients don't seem to think that the medications make them feel better. The World Health Organization (WHO) asserts that by improving medication adherence, we'll be able to solve more issues than we can by a lot of new inventions hitting the market.[95] One way we can achieve this is by utilizing big data from pharmacy transactions to reach out to patients and collaborate with them to support prescription adherence.

CHALLENGES IN BIG DATA

Big data mining within the healthcare industry is in its early stages, so it's common to have areas that can be improved upon. Considering that most healthcare systems went onto an

---

95   World Healthcare Organization. "Adherence to Long-Term Therapies: Evidence for action." (2003).

EMR only in the last three to five years, this growth in big data has been very rapid, so issues are to be expected.

Aside from underutilized data, a major challenge is that the data within most healthcare systems exists in silos. For example, within a large corporation, the finance department has its data, which is in "French" and stored in its own database. The quality assurance department has its data in "Russian," which is again separated into another database. Then an EMR, for example, will be in "Japanese" and completely separate from the other databases. The trend continues across departments and countries. When the CEO requests specific information to improve company efficiency, all the separate departments looking at their separate and isolated data may each have a different response to the same question. These differences are often significant, and drawing accurate conclusions from the data becomes nearly impossible.

To work successfully, healthcare organizations need to break down silos between departments and subscribe to a single data source governed by one set of data definitions. Investing in experienced and qualified data scientists as well as professional grade, standardized data programs will allow for this to happen successfully, ensuring valuable insights in the future.

In the field of big data analytics, people talk about acquiring insights instead of reaching conclusions. We're describing shades of gray as opposed to saying it's a black-and-white conclusion. For instance, as part of current guideline recommendations, children are screened for lead toxicity generally at ages one or two, and those blood lead levels are then reported to the state as well as the CDC. The state or CDC can then plot that data to the child's home address and visualize where lead is toxic in some neighborhoods and where it's maybe okay in others, since the majority of lead comes from the soil or lead paint. Plotting that out, one can make inferences that otherwise would be invisible to us and use this in order to find solutions.

While the data cannot determine whether an individual patient has lead poisoning, it allows me to infer that the patient has a higher risk of being poisoned by lead and that I should monitor more closely as well as provide actionable tools to the parents to reduce lead exposure.

If you recall, Google created Google Flu Trends as an emerging app several years ago, and then it went off the grid. The app monitored search activity for flu-like symptoms, and based on this they were able to predict, with a fair degree of accuracy, flu trends over time. Ultimately however, there were some significant flu epidemics that were missed based on the set of search terms used in the model, so Google Flu Trends was taken off the shelf, though it remains available to researchers.

Companies and individuals are now building on the ideas and technology behind Google Flu Trends. The takeaway here is that using such batches of information helps to create increasingly accurate models. Information sources are growing in volume and variety and not only include search terms in search engines but social media posts such as Twitter and Facebook. The implications of such effective models are endless.

Possibilities Through Big Data

The focus on capturing and recording information directly from patients is new and gaining momentum. The telehealth care that permits physicians and other care providers to treat something like high blood pressure without a single office visit necessitates data collection on blood pressure, time at home, activity level, and so on. The care provider then virtually connects with the patient via phone, email, or message. In situations such as this, asking the patient the right questions is a significant factor in achieving desired results.

With that in mind, we are creating new technologies to support data collection from patients. Take a chronic issue, like asthma, where a patient can feel physically well for a long time and then begin to display symptoms. Most of the time, these early symptoms are mild and resolve, but other times they may progressively deteriorate and lead to an emergency room visit or worse, a hospitalization. Waiting for a clinic appointment is not often an effective alternative.

Now, with new technology, we can provide better solutions for patients. The apps and other technologies we are developing can ask the patient questions once or twice a week and even monitor inhaler usage through Bluetooth connectivity. The patient's responses and inhaler frequency will help determine the best next step. If a patient is feeling more short of breath, experiencing even small changes in breathing, or has developed a new cough, the app can notify the care team that the this patients needs close monitoring and further evaluation. The care team may possibly prescribe additional therapy or reassess treatment or arrange an office visit that day. Such an outcome is significantly better than waiting for the patient's health to really decline before intervening. I'm using asthma as an example, but imagine how significant this type of technology could revolutionize the patient experience and outcome for other illnesses and conditions. We could catch patients early as opposed to waiting for an extreme situation that may be too late to impact without a full-blown hospitalization.

These technologies can also include environmental data so that care providers are aware of the level of humidity, the pollen count, air quality index, and so on. As the physician, I can say, "I'm noticing that when X and Y and Z occur, F happens." The data allows one to make inferences of triggers and factors in order to determine the best preemptive medicine, treatment, or lifestyle change.

The relationship between social networks and big data is also very valuable and holds a lot of potential. Cell phone traffic alone allows us to predict economic output and crime rates in cities across the world. This does not refer to the conversations or words used, but just by looking at the number of calls and the number of people that you call, the duration of calls, the time they start, and so on, the data can predict economic and crime-related activity. This is an example of how big data and social interactions can predict outcomes.

A lot of information can be predicted based on the number of different people you communicate with and the duration of those communications. Since social activities show a tight correlation to one's mood, this data allows us to infer if someone is alone, depressed, isolated, happy, or sad, which, as we know, is often directly correlated with one's health.

As another example, let's look at the differences between a routine pedometer and a Fitbit. A Fitbit is basically a fancy pedometer that tracks your steps. What distinguishes it and makes it more effective than merely tracking steps is that can tie the user to a social network. Research generally shows that people are more likely to do things that they see other people doing, and that most people have some level of competition with friends in their social network. The ability to share your tracking results and to view others' results feeds into these human motivators. It comes as no surprise, then, that research now shows that people have increased activity when using a Fitbit, which is connected to their social network, than when using a pedometer that only tracks their steps. There is value in social networks altering behavior as well as in inferring big data.

BIG DATA CONTROVERSY

The controversies surrounding big data are generally about anonymity and privacy. People may know more about you than you want them to know. For instance, I can buy television data from your cable company, from DirecTV, from Dish, and so on. This means that not only is there a record of how many hours of TV you watch, but also that you like to watch the news and that you like to watch *Game of Thrones* as well as the History Channel. With this information, a company like Amazon will approach you with what they think you'll be interested in purchasing based on your other interests. By inferring data, Amazon and other companies are able to predict purchasing behavior, and as long as they are correct more often than they are incorrect, it's useful information.

While that's an example of direct-to-consumer marketing, there is also direct-to-phenotype marketing. The buying and selling of such data is more extensive than we realize. Much of the time, we don't even know the data exists, much less the transactions that are occurring.

Your healthcare data doesn't go out or get sold to companies the way your shopping and viewing interests do because it's protected health data. Your data from a healthcare system is protected under HIPAA (the Health Insurance Portability and Accountability Act of 1996), so that data cannot be purchased like your DirecTV data or your cable data. Unless a hacker successfully breaks into your healthcare system and steals your data, your information is secure. However, medical record theft is actually one of the biggest sources of cybercrime that exists today on a worldwide basis. There are lots of attacks on systems to try and steal medical data because it turns out to be more valuable than your credit card information.

There are definite benefits to electronic medical data, but the risk is that a sophisticated hacker will be able to break into any system, however protected. Though healthcare data is protected, the main concern remains whether or not our personal information is being shared with others. Unless the information is stolen, it can only be released to a third party with patient permission. For example, if you're seeing Dr. Jones and decide to visit Dr. Smith instead, you'll ask Dr. Jones' office to send your medical records to Dr. Smith's office. The staff with Dr. Jones can only do so after you've signed a consent form allowing the transfer of data. The only time that healthcare provider data can be shared without your consent is in the case of an emergency. If a patient arrives at another hospital for something like a heart attack and is unable to consent to medical information transfer, the medical office will still release information to the hospital as it may allow for better care which may help to save the patient's life.

Big data and gaining inference can also become controversial when it comes to the actions taken based on the information. Genomics, for example, is another big data to source. If a patient's genetic profile suggests that an individual is at increased risk for developing heart disease in their lifetime, then the physician should communicate this to the patient and work on reducing when possible any modifiable risk factors, to reduce that risk. However, if someone were to misuse or misunderstand the information and suggest that the patient needs an invasive heart procedure, that type of behavior is what contributes to controversy around big data or genomics.

The appropriate action would be to state that just because you have an increased risk doesn't mean that you're going to develop a disease, it just necessitates a screening frequency that is different from that of a person less likely to develop heart disease. It all boils down to using the information for reasonable action, instead of placing the patient in additional harm through unnecessary treatment or testing. The physician's role should be to heighten vigilance for that type of patient, not to cause panic.

BENEFITS OF BIG DATA IN HEALTHCARE

I predict that the greatest benefits of using big data analytics in the healthcare industry will be seen in the prevention and management of chronic disease. Returning to our example with asthma, the physician can now predict when the patient's health will potentially deteriorate before it actually happens, or at least at the onset of early symptoms. Chronic diseases, like diabetes or heart failure, are generally with the patient for the rest of his or her life, which means that a multitude of factors influence whether the patient will have a successful day, week, or month. These factors include what's going on in the environment, the people the patient interacts with, diet, and other habitual behaviors. So the more information the care provider can have on all the factors that influence the patient's chronic disease, the more appropriately the care provider can intervene. Something as simple as a phone call from the care provider can make a significant impact on a patient struggling to manage a chronic disease.

I believe that we'll see another large impact from big data in genomics, which will be largely along the same lines as chronic disease because of the significant role that patient behavior plays in wellness. Epigenetics relates to using behavior to actually change your genetic expression. If you are genetically predisposed to high blood pressure but your physician helps you maintain a healthy diet and active lifestyle, you're far less likely to run into issues with high blood pressure and may actually change the way your genes work in your favor. We can use big data about individual behaviors to provide you with insights that you don't currently have. Further, we're able to do this in real time instead of running into health issues and explaining how behavior could have prevented the deterioration.

Big data will change the face of healthcare for physicians as well. It's going to provide insight in terms of decision support that physicians have never had before. Physicians want their patients to be healthy and feel well enough to not need to visit the doctor. The point is that the goal of healthcare, since its inception, is to try to use increasingly better tools in order to accomplish this. The tools that big data provides can be enormously helpful in terms of customizing treatments to each individual.

Considering the benefits from big data ties back to my earlier chapter on precision medicine. Big data will provide us with the ability to increase precision in terms of individual treatment plans, including cancer chemotherapy. Currently, cancer diagnoses are grouped by the source of origin, the organ where the cancer initially grew. This form of categorization holds minimal value, because a unique genetic description of the cancer is actually necessary in order to tailor a unique therapy that will work. The only way we can figure that out is through genomic data, by looking at fifty other people across the globe who have something similar to that genetically, and how they responded to specific types of treatment. That's the ultimate success of big data: knowing what will work for individual patients by having access to all of the needed information.

Essentially, big data is going to make the idea of the average patient obsolete. There's not going to be such a thing as the average patient anymore, just like there's no such thing as the average consumer. When companies provided everyone with the same direct-to-consumer advertising, they created brand recognition. Now, Amazon is looking at personal travel interests and combining that information with the type of shoes and handbags the consumer is shopping for in order to provide specialized suggestions in luggage. Similarly, big data will allow us to reach the point where there is no average patient.

Finally, let's look at the financial benefits of using big data. The recent report from McKinsey & Co. estimates that big data analytics can enable more than $300 billion in savings per year. Big data analytics will take a large portion of expense out of several aspects of healthcare, such as reducing the costs of clinical trials, research and development, genomics analysis, and more.

Let's take a closer look at research and development: If a company produces a new form of chemotherapy in the treatment of ovarian cancer, it would perform a large and expensive trial on these women in hopes of providing a lifesaving benefit. Let's assume the trial is modestly successful and yields a 15 percent reduction in death. That's great for the women who benefited but not so great for the many others who did not. Now what if we evaluated the genetic makeup of those who survived and performed a smaller trial on women who match that genetic profile. We may now see a 90 percent reduction in death, which is incredible, and now know that this is the treatment of choice for ovarian cancer patients with this unique genetic profile. The remaining women who would have never benefited would choose a different and more likely effective treatment regimen.

The point is that the same therapy applied generally to patients with ovarian cancer may statistically show low success rates and the therapy will be deemed not beneficial enough to continue. So the women with the specific phenotype that would benefit from the therapy do not have access to it. Applied correctly, the same therapy can show a 90 percent or more success rate. It will reduce the number of people the therapy needs to be administered to in order to see a benefit. Overall, it reduces costs, increases efficiency, and, most importantly, provides the correct treatment to the right patient.

Big data will provide precision-focused research and development as well, which will further drop healthcare costs. Money will need to be invested into advanced analytics in order to reach accurate conclusions, but that will yield a very positive ROI.

The future of the healthcare industry is exciting because data is increasing at unfathomable rates. Data on blood pressure, heart rate, temperature, can all be done in a hospital without a nurse—only a device collecting data from a patient and automatically sending the information to an EMR. As big data continues to progress, it will get to the point of monitoring patients at home, with their permission of course. Imagine what that means for elderly care: we can collect data on how much someone is moving around at home, how many times their front door opens, the number of times the toilet flushes, and so on. We can easily determine if patients are eating enough, getting out, able to care for themselves, or if they're in need of help perhaps before they may realize they need help. This is only an example of the ways in which big data will help the healthcare industry provide individualized care for people who will truly benefit from it.

Big data is relatively new and progressing at unprecedented rates. There are definitely limitations and challenges in the current collection and use of big data within the healthcare industry, but we are seeing improvements regularly. The potential benefits of big data within the healthcare industry are exponential.

CHAPTER 9

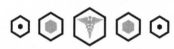

Reengineering Healthcare Delivery Beyond Patching a Broken System

Earlier this year, Bernard Tyson, CEO of Kaiser Permanente, tweeted, "If I was redesigning Kaiser Permanente today, I would start with technology. Everything else follows." Tyson gets it: technology can help reengineer our healthcare system to save more lives and improve quality of life for more people while decreasing overall healthcare costs. Our current healthcare system was established over one hundred years ago, when the public had very different needs than today, but the system has not evolved to the point of effectively managing the chronic diseases and illnesses that are becoming increasingly prevalent. Kaiser is a large delivery system that's also the insurer—they realize that they can achieve greater financial benefits down the line, by investing in preventive patient care now. That is precisely why Tyson recognizes the significance of strategically using technology so that it can enable immediate, evidence-based, and results-focused preventive care.

In 2012 the New England Journal of Medicine published "The Burden of Disease and the Changing Task of Medicine." While the article outlines several relevant points, one line stands out: "In many respects, our medical systems are best suited to diseases of the past, not those of the present or future." The primary diseases of the past were episodic and acute, so that's what the healthcare system is built on. We're built to be able to analyze severe symptoms, such as coughing up blood, and make the diagnosis of TB or pneumonia, treat the patient for the specific issue, and, once cured, there's no further follow-up. While urgent and episodic patient needs will always exist, that approach should be a component of our system, not the basis of our current healthcare system. We now need to create an entirely different system in order to be able to manage the prevailing issues of the public today.

The majority of ailments affecting the public today are chronic diseases and, often, multiple chronic diseases per patient. This proposes a different burden on the healthcare system as opposed to the episodic and primarily infectious diseases that took place in the 1900s. The disease burden that takes place today is primarily chronic diseases. While they most certainly can be life threatening, they are not episodic and must be managed on a continual basis. Yet our healthcare delivery system was built on the former burden, not the latter. Another article in the New England Journal of Medicine, "The Quality of Health Care Delivered to Adults in the United States," conducted research on the level of healthcare provided to a specific group of adults in the United States and found that under 55 percent of participants received the evidence-based recommended care.

We now have an entirely different disease burden that's affecting our population, and we need a different system to be able to manage chronic ailments that generally stem from behavioral and lifestyle choices. The level of attention, detail, and data that is necessary for effectively monitoring and managing chronic disease was previously impossible. Advancements in technology today now make it possible for patients and physicians to work together toward health goals, and for physicians to effectively reach out to and even treat people without geographic restraints. The possibilities are limitless, but we need to reengineer the healthcare system into one that fully integrates the appropriate technologies in order to optimize patient care.

CHALLENGES TO REENGINEERING HEALTHCARE

The challenge of reengineering our current healthcare system isn't necessarily a lack of resources, but the lack of a unified vision and purpose for the medical industry. While Kaiser's Tyson is promoting the use of technology, other thought leaders are perpetuating outdated approaches to healthcare. Recently, James L. Madara, the CEO of the American Medical Association, made several statements about current trends in the industry. Firstly, he stated that mobile health technology has no real medicinal value. Madara also stated that he doesn't personally use an electronic medical record (EMR). His overall statement was that advancements such as telemedicine, digital health, and so on don't adequately foster a doctor-patient relationship. This statement is detrimental to progress in the healthcare industry because the prime directive is not to develop relationships, but to promote the health and wellbeing of the public. Our goal is to ensure that our patients' health is managed in the most effective and efficient way possible. The end result is people living to their greatest health potential while decreasing personal and total healthcare expenditures. These are the prime objectives of healthcare, not building relationships between doctors and patients.

Madara's perspective and initiative is no longer relevant if the healthcare industry is to meet the needs of today's public. Promoting electronic data, data sharing, and digital health for expediency and increased accuracy should be a priority, but Madara's statements serve as blockades to such progress. The reality is that EMRs and healthcare-centric technologies are already integrated into our system, so we are presently beginning to see their benefits, but not yet reaching their full potential. Current data shows that many people are sick because of what they eat and/or because they are physically inactive. Still, our healthcare system isn't designed to counter these behavioral issues and to approach the chronic ailments that they give rise to. The majority of thought leaders in the industry, academics, scholars, data scientists, and so on, are confirming these trends and calling for the reengineering of our current system. The statements given by CEO of the AMA are shocking in how greatly they differ from what the research shows. While it is unclear whether the statements are representative of most of the members of that organization, true progress will not be possible until we have a unified vision and objective.

If Madara is representing mainstream healthcare, or at least a portion of mainstream healthcare, we clearly have a system in need of great repairs and we have a long way to go. Currently, our systems sets it up so that physicians diagnose something like diabetes, prescribe medication, give recommended lifestyle changes, then schedule a follow-up visit six months later. What if in six months the patient is doing very well? The patient would visit the physician, explain lifestyle and activities since the last visit, pay for the office visit or copay, parking, and so on, and that's the entirety of the visit. It has no value for the patient, and the physician merely notes the visit. That's it. The only thing that that visit works toward is developing more of a connection, or relationship, between the physician and the patient.

Legacy processes and IT systems are also impediments to reengineering the healthcare system. Most organizations currently have some kind of IT system in place, but those systems age rather quickly. Instead of replacing the legacy system, which can be really expensive, organizations add more technology in patch-type fixes. That's a solution for the short-term, but in the long-term we have ineffective technology that can't meet the needs of health organizations.

Several years ago, most hospitals had either rudimentary IT systems or no IT system at all, which didn't allow for comprehensive care. The High Tech Act was implemented as part of the Accountable Care Act, which basically created financial incentives for hospitals and physician's offices to use new technology that had to be EMR certified. This allowed for rapid and swift change in the field.

The one downfall to the governmental initiative to move the use of technology forward in the healthcare industry is that the offices, hospitals, and organizations implemented different programs and systems written in different codes and languages. Instead of everyone speaking one language and communicating with each other, we have the equivalent of French, German, Spanish, Japanese, and so on. These systems don't have interoperability, which is fine if patients don't need any services or visits to anyone outside of a single healthcare system. When a patient goes to another hospital, physician, or surgeon, their information doesn't always transfer, which becomes costly and causes delays to receiving quality care and sometimes duplication of services or worse.

A solution to the issue of multiple IT systems in the healthcare industry that cannot communicate with each other is patient-oriented systems—a personal health information system for each patient. Down the line everyone will ultimately have their own individual health information system, probably made by a large digital company. The point is that patients will own 100 percent of their data in their personal system, and the patient will give the physician a portal into his or her system so that the doctor can see all the necessary information. That will be an important and necessary step in the evolution of the healthcare system.

AUTOMATED CARE

In 2012, the *New England Journal of Medicine* published an article, "Automated Hovering in Healthcare—Watching Over the 5000 Hours." In summation, the research in this article focuses on the fact that for the 5,000 hours each year that you are engaging in work, sleep, home, and everything else, you are not seeing your doctor. It's not that you need to see your doctor constantly, but having an automated hovering device will enable data collection on your health and activities that will enable the best preventive care possible. Such a process would not be something that you would have to manually work with or constantly think about, which makes it accessible for most people.

The automated hovering service would notify your doctor that you're well and save you the hassle of going into the office for a routine follow-up visit. Likewise, it would allow your doctor to reach out anytime there was a possible reason for concern and schedule the appointment as necessary, regardless of the amount of time that had passed since the last visit. We don't quite know the optimal frequency of visits, but if the goal is to maintain health, we can personalize the means, whether the visit is three years or six weeks apart, and that will allow us to achieve our goal of meaningful health interactions. As of now, we often see patients who don't need to be seen, and then wait until some patients who are in need fall off the edge, ultimately being seen in the emergency room or urgent care. Instead of focusing on relationships, we need to ask ourselves, and each other, how we can develop a system that's not just based on a doctor that can do things and serve as the only resource from the healthcare perspective, but based on patient-doctor partnerships that target lifestyle and behavior changes and enable optimal health.

The most common chronic disease in the world, hypertension (also known as high blood pressure), is also the most common chronic disease in the United States: one out of every three adults has high blood pressure. Uncontrolled hypertension leads to dementia, heart disease, and stroke. It's also the second leading cause of kidney failure, not to mention other things like eye disease. Uncontrolled hypertension is extremely destructive to the body and its effects are seen in all organs, and costs huge sums of money. Unfortunately, one out of every six people in the United States, or half of those with hypertension, has *uncontrolled* hypertension.

It's ridiculous that in this day and age a controllable condition remains extremely rampant and destructive; it's an epidemic. This is one area that will see significant improvements if the overall healthcare system is reengineered. Moreover, we don't need thousands of doctors to do it. Clinical pharmacists, health coaches, data scientists, and so on can contribute to effectively controlling hypertension for the majority of people in the United States. Hypertension is something that can be corrected, controlled, and managed. We don't need new medicines. We don't need to conduct costly and invasive procedures. We just need the patient's help. Moreover, depending on the level of motivation on the patient's part, there are many things that people can do to control hypertension while lessening or even completely cutting drugs. We need a system that empowers people to change so that instead of thinking that they have no control, they take action to manage their health. We've developed such a system at Ochsner, where 71 percent of patients with previously uncontrolled hypertension achieve complete control within ninety days. We accomplish this by engaging patients in their own care, and by use of real-time data coming directly from the patient's home to their doctor's office. It results in dramatically better outcomes that are more convenient for patients and at a lower cost.

Other research shows that more than half of the dollars spent in healthcare within the United States are actually spent on a very small percentage of the population, close to about 5 percent.[96] This research is not necessarily focusing on the costs of maintaining healthcare needs at the end of life, but on monies spent on people who have multiple chronic diseases, for example, someone with hypertension, diabetes, and chronic obstructive pulmonary disease (COPD). The truth is that the more diseases a person has, the shorter that person's life expectancy, but there is a lot of money spent on managing the symptoms and effects for as long as possible.

A common situation in the hospital setting is with older people who have one or more conditions that have compromised their health and quality of life until they have become hospitalized with a very small chance of survival. Imagine someone in the intensive care unit, on a ventilator, her family and loved ones in the waiting room, and her blood pressure falling. In order to

---

96   Weissman, Jordan. "5% of Americans Made Up 50% of U.S. Health Care Spending." The Atlantic. January 13, 2012. https://www. theatlantic.com/business/archive/2012/01/5-of-americans-made-up-of-us-health-care-spending/251402/.

maintain the patient's blood pressure, the physician will have to put in an expensive balloon pump, which is uncomfortable, but it's going to keep her alive for a few days. Unless the patient has already written a "Do Not Resuscitate" clause within a living will, the physician cannot make the decision of whether or not to continue the costly and invasive treatments as long as she is alive. At this point the physician approaches the family, and generally the decision is that the patient has suffered enough and that nature should take its course. There are other families who decide that it's better to keep the patient alive regardless of the consequences and costs, and in these instances a lot of money is spent on the last days and weeks of life. Some of it is done intelligently, but tangible consequences to the spending could inform decisions differently.

THE FREE MARKET

In terms of reengineering healthcare delivery, the questions we should be asking are: Who is going to set healthcare policy priorities? Who has the right to set healthcare priorities? The public should decide the priorities in healthcare policies, and the only way to ensure that that happens is through the free market. The current problem is that the healthcare system is not paying attention to what the free market is communicating. The public is dying from chronic disease complications, yet thought leaders in the healthcare industry are focusing on doctor-patient relationships and putting up barricades to electronic health records and digital real-time solutions. Such leaders do not understand the disease burden of the public, and they are not trying to create an appropriately responsive system. It is going to take a disruption to the current system and way of thought to create real change. Healthcare-centric start-ups combining technology, social media, and data science are currently working on the tools and resources that are going to create an effective disruption.

The public today is searching the Internet for the information they need: detailed medical data, access to multiple opinions, and so on. This empowers patients to challenge the doctor's opinions, which breaks down the patriarchal approach of the traditional doctor-patient relationship. What some are not realizing is that asking for alternatives and questioning the doctor's recommendations is actually going to be a benefit to healthcare. On the same note, high deductibles will also be beneficial because they drive patients to question things just as they would with any other advisor, expertise, or services that are paid for. When patients are more engaged in the process and financial consequences, they will be empowered to demand the quality care and attention they need and deserve. The free market will then determine the priorities by virtue of the needs of what people want, as opposed to coming from the top down.

Looping back to the point of personal health information systems, the vast majority of consumers want full access to their medical records while the majority of doctors want to give patients limited access to their health information. The important thing to keep in mind is that there is only person in the entire equation who has an interest in making sure the information in the medical record is accurate; that is the patient. Physicians will make mistakes, and incorrect data may be entered, but the patient is the one invested enough to look, double-check, and speak up when things are not right. Giving the patient full control will allow the market to determine healthcare priorities, and companies that meet the market demand will succeed. There will be companies that don't even exist yet that are going to change the way people receive healthcare.

The combination of technology, consumerism, and high-deductible health insurance, will create a perfect storm that will reengineer the healthcare system. What capitalism has taught us is that paying more for an item or service increases expectations and demands. Any healthcare delivery system that is not embracing these changes is clearly going to lose. Moreover, anybody that is invested too heavily in bricks and mortar won't be able to stay relevant as we reengineer healthcare.

Now that the healthcare system is moving toward EMRs, there's suddenly an abundance of data and information. Companies and consumers don't know what to do with all of the data, though there is a lot of value in that data. Value in terms of saving lives, making discoveries, and driving improvement. Next, we'll see a rise in analytical systems that will be able to manage data. Over 90 percent of the world's data, not just in healthcare, but overall data, has accrued in the last two years. If this is also true for healthcare systems, instead of paper archives and documentation, we now have an enormous amount of untapped digital information. There are health systems that are not building adequate analytic capabilities to be able to deal with their accumulating data, and there are health systems that are trying to do that well. The future will be data-driven learning and analytics that not only create and sustain economies, but also are the safest and most efficient option yielding the highest quality for the patient. This is all in the works now.

Many people are wondering whether we are moving fast enough to reengineer healthcare. That is an ironic question because the answer is probably no, even though we are moving very fast. The pace of change for all things, besides healthcare, is incredibly fast and getting faster. So while the healthcare industry is making huge strides and progressing, from the patient perspective, we just aren't moving fast enough.

Eventually everything is going to be on-demand—where you can schedule anything you want: physician visits, phone calls, specialist visits, and so on will be available around the clock. Here's information about you when you need it at the time you need it. That's what technology can do, create a healthcare system around the patient and build resources from that. Technology will enable and empower patients to get the care they need when they need it, and in the way that is most suitable to them. If I were to rebuild healthcare, I, like Bernard Tyson wouldn't build what we have today. I would build a system that can unobtrusively monitor your health and alert you and your team when you may need to do something. When you need care, you would have it in the time and place of your choosing. Similarly, you would know what things costs and fully understand the quality of care and patient ratings of any number of available healthcare providers.

Within the healthcare industry, we are already practicing a great deal of telemedicine. For example, a patient suffering a stroke can now receive care from a stroke specialist located hundreds of miles away, leading to life-saving measures available to almost anyone in any zip code.

If the number one priority for the healthcare system is the doctor-patient relationship, then we are not going to live up to our full potential, and that patient with a stroke may not survive. If, however, our number one priority is the health and wellness of individuals, we will innovate in every way possible to ensure that we are saving lives and improving health. Physicians will always work towards putting their patients first. The question then becomes whether we are confident in our ability to execute and achieve these goals. Do we have the resources to pull this off? If not, let's start looking into what we need and how we can get it. Technology integration will be a key to creating that level of effectiveness within the healthcare industry.

CHAPTER 10

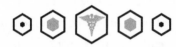

The Future of Healthcare

T he future of medicine is brighter than most believe. The concern has generally been: How will the healthcare industry advance life-saving, economically feasible healthcare focused on managing chronic disease? As I have discussed throughout the book, this is not only possible, but it is actually the direction our healthcare industry is headed. A major component of achieving this goal is the movement toward precision medicine, which refers to the healthcare industry embracing individualized care and moving away from the current method of standardized treatments for patients.

In medicine today, physicians are treating everyone with a specific disease or condition with one particular therapy, though it may only benefit a relatively small percentage of patients. The physician cannot know which patients will benefit from the treatment and which won't, so each patient pays the premium and receives treatment that in many cases won't help. It's similar to a lottery system.

With precision medicine, the physician can pinpoint who will benefit from which treatment and can then prescribe a different treatment for the others, or refer them out to specialists who can help. Essentially, precision medicine is going to be a win for everyone involved: it will be a more cost-effective and efficient method of treatment.

New technologies and advancements in diagnosis and treatment enhance our ability to administer and implement precision medicine. Nanotechnology, organ-on-a-chip, and liquid biopsy are a few examples of such possibilities. These are all tools that are highly cost-effective because we no longer have to treat one hundred people to heal only a small percentage. Such innovations and developments allow physicians to provide the right therapy to the right person in the right way.

CUTTING-EDGE TECHNOLOGIES

Nanotechnology, for instance, works at the individual atom level and makes it possible for us to find the exact location of a growth and deliver therapy (such as radiation or drug therapy) only to that spot. The end result is a more precise therapy, which means fewer visits, copays, and so on, all while creating a greater likelihood of full recovery without severe side effects.

The cognitive computer is another example of technology that will allow us to make better decisions in real time so that we're using more appropriate therapies while minimizing the possibility of error. IBM's Watson computer analytically processes disparate data to help curate information and offer tailored care. Computers such as Watson can actually come up with a hypothesis based on its independent evaluation of data. Even more exciting are the possibilities that may come from quantum computing, which are next generation computers that replace standard "bits" of data (only in one of two states, "0" or "1") with quantum bits or qubits of data (which can have a value of "0," "1," or both "0" and "1" at the same time). Quantum computing is much more powerful than conventional computing and has the possibility of creating major breakthroughs in medicine and artificial intelligence, and this is only one to two years away. Once this technology becomes more fully integrated into our healthcare system, it will fundamentally change how we diagnose and treat patients.

The liquid biopsy, which refers to analyzing blood rather than tissue for tumor cells, will also revolutionize healthcare in terms of being able to detect small changes before a disease progresses and while it may still be manageable. In terms of genomes or micro-RNA that's being released, we can detect extremely small changes at an earlier stage and help the patient heal more quickly than we can at a later stage when symptoms are present.

Similarly, a new technology called organ-on-a-chip will fundamentally change drug development and drug therapy, improving the time and costs related to receiving necessary therapies. An organ-on-a-chip contains a cell culture of a human organ embedded on a chip that simulates the actual functioning of the human organ. By acting as an artificial organ, drugs and other novel therapies can be tested easily and quickly without involving human subjects. Getting drug therapies out to market faster will make it less expensive for entities to develop new products and test new interventions. Rather than having to conduct tests and efficacy trials with humans, drug companies can use an organ-on-a-chip to run less costly and less risky tests. If the drug therapy passes based on the organ-on-a-chip test, the drug can be deemed ready to go on the market. This will lead to faster development of more effective therapies.

It won't be long before these technologies become mainstream. The lung-on-a-chip already exists. The device functions like a computer but acts like a human lung and is able to oxygenate blood that passes through it. Once technology like lung-on-a-chip is in mass production, companies will be able to test any compound they are working quickly and inexpensively.

Liquid biopsy is also already available, though it is not very widespread. There are only a couple of companies that offer the procedure right now. Several companies and research organizations are working on developing and implementing the liquid biopsy, and we'll soon see it on a much broader scale.

All of these innovations are in their infancy, but they do exist. Within the next few years, these technologies will become much more mainstream. The idea is that there are certain types of decisions and diagnoses that well-designed computer systems can make more accurately than humans can.

Each of these cutting-edge technologies is contributing to more precise methods of diagnosis and treatment. The more accurate the diagnoses and treatments are, the more cost-effective the overall process will be for patients, physicians, and insurance companies. Essentially, precision medicine creates a more sustainable and beneficial healthcare environment for everyone involved.

BIG DATA

As we previously discussed, big data is going to be extremely valuable, but it will be an ongoing issue as well. There are several challenges that the healthcare industry will have to address. Number one, obviously, is that there is an overwhelming amount of information out there. It's time-consuming for any kind of computer to sort and interpret the data. There are millions of papers that Watson, for example, has already gone through, and it continues to be fed research on a regular basis.

The second major challenge to big data is enabling cognitive computers to interpret nuance—something that humans can do inherently. This has proven to be a difficult challenge to overcome. If I, as the physician, am writing in a note about sleepiness, am I trying to get you to sleep? Are you getting too much sleep? Are you having difficulty with sleep? Is it a side effect of the medicine? There's a lot of nuance just with that one word, and the cognitive computer must correctly interpret the context and implications. This is still a work in progress.

The other main concern with big data is security. We need to continue to find more effective methods of protecting medical data. Is your information going to remain private? Is it information that can get out to an insurance company, employer, or any other entity? A current issue our society is dealing with, on several levels, is that data and private information is constantly being leaked or hacked into.

If I don't want people to know that I have cardiovascular issues or a terminal illness, I won't want this information stored in an unsafe space. Currently, personal medical information has to go through several algorithms for data mining and storage. This means that it's not being held on a piece of paper locked in a vault in a hospital. Creating appropriate levels of security is a significant challenge facing big data, which we need to reconcile before we can fully reap the benefits of big data and the healthcare industry.

As we discussed previously, the healthcare industry is moving toward an outcome-based model, so quantitative evidence will be attached to the payment of services provided. That's one area where big data comes in. The ability to interpret and analyze large amounts of information in terms of patient healthcare and history will provide valuable insights into what's working and what's not. We need to be responsible for our outcomes so that professionals who achieve positive outcomes succeed and those who don't are either marginalized or given the opportunity to improve. Healthcare, in the future, will be purely outcome-based. Big data and the analytics that come from it can ensure that the healthcare industry achieves this improved model of care.

CHRONIC DISEASE AND DATA COLLECTION

The healthcare industry has made significant improvements in terms of chronic disease management. Chronic disease is going to require a continuous model of care, observation, data collection, and delivery as opposed to the current episodic model of care. Technology and big data are headed in the direction where sustainable and effective chronic disease management is now becoming a possibility.

Diabetes management, for example, will completely evolve. The physician can collect data on your blood sugar levels multiple times throughout the day—from twenty to one hundred times—whatever is necessary. All of this information will be possible without even sticking your finger with a needle because the information is continuously assessed through technology that's either implanted or worn. Similarly, the therapy you receive is continuously assessed and monitored. In this way, you receive what you need when you need it, instead of visiting your physician once every six months, waiting for test results, then deciding if any changes are needed.

A major component to the success of using data to manage chronic disease is ensuring that the data collection is safe and does not interfere with any other tasks. It won't work if the patient has to stop every hour and interact with the technology in order for it to collect data.

This level of technology integration can only happen if it collects data passively, without requiring the patient to be aware of it at all times, similar to the Fitbit and Apple Watch. Even your cell phone collects data without you noticing. Every time you have your cell phone on, it knows where you are and if you're moving. It also knows when you talk and who you talk to. This is an enormous amount of information that is continuously collected, all under the radar of the consumer.

Data collection and chronic disease management will become mainstream once we have a solid method of interpreting this volume of data. That will enable us to make important decisions about care delivery and then implement those decisions quickly and effectively. Managing chronic disease in this manner will be highly effective, especially in comparison to current practices. The fact that data collection on chronic disease currently takes place once in every three to four months proves the inefficiency of our process. It takes over six months to make a decision on the appropriate therapy and all the while the data is changing by the minute.

The technology is already there; we just need to take it a few steps further. I'm talking about technology that collects health information from clothing, nanosensors, or any other unobtrusive device. These devices will have the ability to pick up on a single cancer cell the day it appears. At that point the patient can have immediate intervention that's potentially as simple as a pill and without side effects. Potentially there will be no need for chemotherapy or radiation therapy. That's the power of data collection in real time.

The future of healthcare will further evolve so that a heart attack can be detected up to seventy-two hours before it occurs (a time when we already know that events are beginning to take place). The patient can then receive a message to go to the hospital for a full exam and any necessary therapy. The future of data technology will have a powerful impact on the field of healthcare and on the longevity of humans.

At the Genetic Level

In the future, medicine won't focus on treating the symptoms of disease, but on actually curing the disease. It's important to keep in mind that not every illness or disease is genetic. We are also battling epigenetic issues. A genetic issue relates to the genes you receive from your parents. Epigenetic issues relate to how you alter those genes based on your lifestyle, which includes where you live, what you do for a living, how active you are, whom you associate with, and so on. Research has only just begun to scratch the surface of how much power we really have at an epigenetic level.

Many people have been looking at their genes as though they were written in stone. In fact, you're a permeable organism and the environment changes your genetic expression on a weekly, or even daily, basis. All of this change takes place based on what you do, whom you are with, and how you feel. Research shows us a very different way of looking at epigenetics, and it's empowering.

While the future of healthcare is evolving and bringing preventive care to the forefront, I'm not certain that we are going to be able to cure illness and disease via genetics alone. It's not so much an issue of technology, but rather of human behavior. While we can devise and adapt new technology, human behavior is much more difficult to change.

There's also the matter of ethics. For instance, clustered regularly interspaced short palindromic repeats, (CRISPR), is a tremendous development, but it is also the source of much ethical debate.

With CRISPR, parents could pick genetic features for their unborn children. CRISPR has the potential of going into the genes and deleting problem areas while also inserting desirable traits, such as height. This technology has been tried on bacteria and other similar organisms with success, but it hasn't been successfully deployed on a human being yet and ethics has everything to do with it.

CRISPR could prevent devastating conditions such as cystic fibrosis, but for each life the mechanism could save, we would also open the door for "designer babies." And we simply don't know how dire the impact of genetically manipulated humans could be on the rest of humanity.

I personally would want to do everything that I could to cure a genetic disease, but where are my limits? If it is possible, the human race needs to be in agreement on specific limitations. Then, we need to hold ourselves accountable to those boundaries. This is science and it's going to advance, which isn't inherently bad, but there are moral issues that must be discussed.

THE SOCIAL FACTOR

The healthcare industry typically has a relatively narrow view of health. When you visit the doctor, he takes your stats, reviews your medical history, and then perhaps runs a blood test. The physician then comes up with a package of diagnoses and therapies, and sends you on your way. We don't take into account a lot of these other very impactful issues, like social determinants, that have nothing to do with our classic model of physician-patient interaction but are nevertheless very important, particularly if you have a chronic condition.

Access to care, health literacy, diet, behavior, and social interactions are major components of successfully managing or healing from disease. As healthcare evolves, these factors are going to be more significant in treatment plans and diagnoses. A broader view of you as a "patient" is going to be necessary, and health systems will take the time to discover this information when we move to an outcome-based model of care. Our traditional method of care may be sufficient in a fee-for-service model, but a broader view of health determinants will be needed to be successful in an outcome-based model.

In earlier chapters I discussed the impact of social isolation, and this has been shown to affect your genes and your risk of disease including heart attack and stroke. So your social environment plays a big role in your health. As physicians, we need to be able to identify patient social support systems, and help patients find methods of managing their social lives in ways conducive to their health.

The people we spend time with make a significant difference in our health and wellbeing, and our social networks are extremely influential for us. If our friends smoke, it's much more likely that we are going to smoke. If the people we spend the most time with are overweight, our chances of being overweight increase. Similarly, if we spend time with people who exercise, we are more likely to exercise ourselves. The people you spend time with alter your genetic expression and you alter theirs.

Your genes express different compounds as a result of these activities. Take the honeybee and Africanized honeybee (also known as "killer bee") for example. Though from the same species, the honeybee and Africanized honeybee are actually quite different. For example, if you went to a honeybee nest and hit it, there might be a couple of thousand bees in the nest and about a hundred of them would come after you to get you to leave them alone. If you went to an Africanized honeybee nest and hit it, you would likely have a thousand bees coming after you ready to kill you. The Africanized honeybee is much more aggressive and has actually evolved to look more intimidating as well.

The experiment for the research was simple: scientists took larvae from standard honeybees and placed them in an Africanized honeybee hive. Bees are known to be very friendly, in the sense that they'll take others in as long as they're not threatening, so the larvae were accepted into the hive. The researchers observed the genetic profiles of the honeybees at birth, then again a month later, two months, three months, and so on. The honeybees were easy to track because the genetic expression of honeybees and Africanized honeybees are quite different.

Researchers found that the larvae, even though they were genetically honeybees, became Africanized. Their whole genetic profile changed, so that they looked and acted like the Africanized honeybees. This research supports the claim that our genetic expression is permeable depending upon factors such as our social environment.

As a physician, there are ways I can collect chronic disease, behavior, and habit information from a patient without having to actually ask for the information. Often, it's these seemingly minor behaviors and habits that make a big difference. We need to improve communication between physicians and patients, while also being able to collect data on behaviors that significantly impact health.

● ⬡ ●

We are permeable, and the impact of others on us, and our impact on others, hold immense potential for the future of healthcare. Incorporating behavioral and social factors into our model of healthcare will significantly enhance our ability to treat chronic disease and genetic issues at a preventive level. Though these components are not yet prevalent in our healthcare model, the evolution and incorporation of progressing technologies are ensuring that it is a possibility in the near future. This will be true precision medicine in practice.

The amount of data that new technologies enable us to collect and analyze allows us insight into our genetic, biologic, and behavioral profile so that we can recognize issues as they begin to develop. Precision medicine will not just be the right therapy for the right person, but it will also come at the right time. Once we are able to detect alterations at the cellular level, our prescribed therapies will be as simple and noninvasive as doing yoga or walking for forty-five minutes a day. Preventive care that also creates social support is even better, as it incorporates social influence into behavioral change: do yoga with a group of people instead of doing it by yourself. We can then check again three months later and see if the exercise is helping or if we need to pursue other avenues of healing.

Precision medicine is preventive care at its best. Data collection and cutting-edge technology will allow us to actually build stronger social networks and manage disease before troubling symptoms arise. Moreover, all of this progress will actually lower costs and help patients, care providers, and insurance agencies save money.

While, as with all things, there are concerns and variables, the future of healthcare is extremely promising.

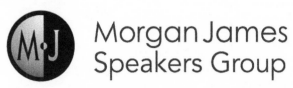

Morgan James
Speakers Group

www.TheMorganJamesSpeakersGroup.com

We connect Morgan James published authors with live and online events and audiences who will benefit from their expertise.

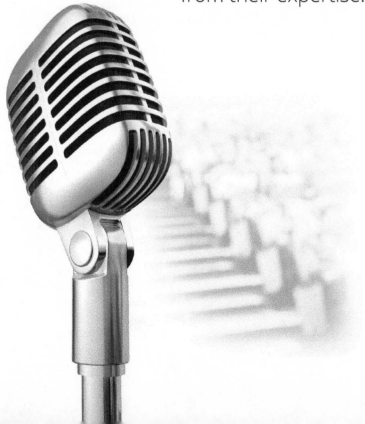

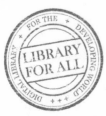